SUSAN S

DARKENED
LIGHT

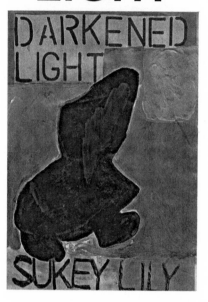

BY SUSAN SPLAINE

'One million people commit suicide every year'
The World Health Organization

SUSAN SPLAINE

Published by
Chipmunkapublishing
PO Box 6872
Brentwood
Essex CM13 1ZT
United Kingdom

http://www.chipmunkapublishing.com

Proof-read by John Matthews

INTRODUCTION

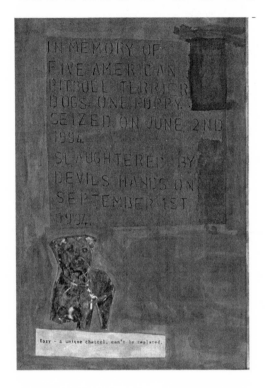

IN MEMORY OF
FIVE AMERICAN
PITBULL TERRIER
DOGS, ONE PUPPY,
SEIZED ON JUNE 2ND
1994.

SLAUGHTERED BY
DEVILS HANDS ON
SEPTEMBER 1ST
1994.

Roxy - a unique chattel, can't be replaced.

SUSAN SPLAINE

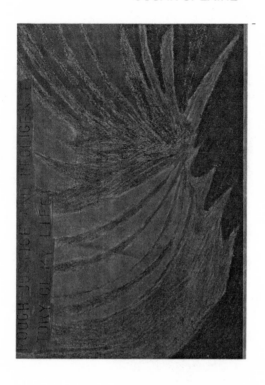

DARKENED LIGHT

Foreword

I have changed people's names and also changed my own name. I have changed the names of supported accommodation hospitals and a psychiatric institution where I have lived for three years.

I want to dedicate my book to my beloved pet Roxy. The police seized her from me in June ninety-ninety-six just because she was a Pit bull. I doted on her and I am sure she was smitten with me because of the love she gave to me. I hit rock bottom and got lost in the darkness because of too many black clouds. Troubled times, unhappiness and uncertainty drained me. I escaped into fantasy because life seemed hazy. Anger came to the surface resulting in resentment. I committed my thoughts to paper. I felt the need for comfort but did not listen to anybody who was sympathetic. The one relationship I had with Milton became strained and deteriorated. I felt as if my lonely life was not worth living.

I have lost my way because of too many black clouds. On the road to nowhere because I was not sure where I was heading. I felt as if I am in the middle of nowhere surrounded by fog because of misfortune and insecurity. From ninety-ninety four to ninety-ninety six it seemed as if day-to-day troubles, traumas were looming over the horizon.

SUSAN SPLAINE

It was not hurting games people played with me. I went to the same places on the board where somebody else was at who intended to bring me harm. My emotions played with because of bad experiences. I felt cheated even though nobody gained victory. The dice rolled without anybody but me looking back.

In life, there is so much traveling and diversity reaching for the stars the skies the limit. I climbed mountains when tumbled down fell flat on my face I felt empty because of blank spaces. Launching new ideas and overcoming obstacles and hindrances should get me onto the road to happiness. Gaps in my life should get smaller when I remember times that do not hurt but please.

The animated wacky world inside my imagination inspired me to draw images for my book. I doodled, colored in the picture and saw imagery that is a form of expression. I have not just described how I feel using words like angry, sad, agitated, irritated and so on. I looked ahead to new horizons with renewal hope and confidence. I kept faith

On my journey, I have found where I blended in. Expressing myself in my book, I have unblocked repressive feelings and memories. On my misfortunes, I built myself back up because I do not live in the past.

DARKENED LIGHT

In ninety-ninety six I listened to George Michael's 'Older' album. I imagined life as a fortune journey because an image came into my mind of bunny rabbits running up hilltops, children flying kites, people having picnics beside a lake. In the far distance, I could see a mountaintop and a light shining down above it. The landscape is where I will shine because of a bright future. When I reach the summit, the light will disappear behind the clouds. I have drawn scattered pieces, pictures for each chapter because of big gaps in life, shadows and clouds needed to drift out of sight. I awaited for my good luck stars to fall down from the sky. Looking up at the purple starlit night waiting for scattered pieces to fall down from the sky and slot into place.

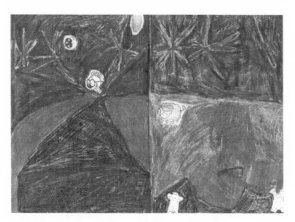

I found a sparkling fallen star.
I lost something precious to me.
My star did not fill in that gap in my life.

When morning broke the blue skies turned grey and black clouds.
I enclosed myself into a field for a few weeks.
There were trees with plenty of foliage for shelter and bearing fruit.
The storm blew down my tree.

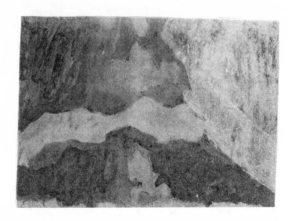

Climbing hills could not get away from worries and troubles.
Personal dilemmas and doubts troubled me underwent pain and severe unhappiness.
Marshland walked across became stuck in the mud.
The river was large and stormy with clear waters.
It took a while but managed to find my way back to dry territory.
Floated safely to shore because came to an expanse of water.

Green countryside surrounded me.
The landscape was a barren one without any trees or flowers.

DARKENED LIGHT

I went through a dark sunless valley with cultivated fields in it.
There was not any shelter from the bitterly cold wind despaired every time that it rained.

On occasion, a pleasant light breeze blew against me.
My hands were cold and my legs were feeling cold.

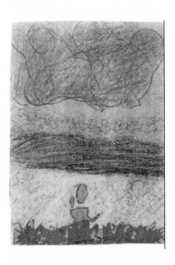

Walking down country lanes got frightening.
I felt the need for solitude and shelter.
The suns light and rays were behind the thunderclouds.
Thunderstorms flash lightning shortly turned day into night.
Thunder and lightning struck everywhere.
Everything struck by lightning all the houses, mountains and hilltops.

It poured down with rain at night and during the day.

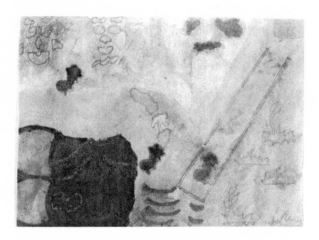

In the floods I managed to keep my head above water.
A man and woman came along and rescued me.
They enlist me getting out off the darkness back into the light.
My intentions will receive there own reward desired to escape craved new experiences.

DARKENED LIGHT

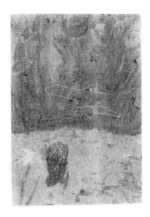

I got onto a moored seaplane to earthly paradise.
Looking down from the seaplane window, I could see shores of body of water.
It was a difficult conquest starting afresh and reforming myself.
I had considerable initiative.
I felt the need to recover some of the freshness and vitality, which had been missing from my life for so long.

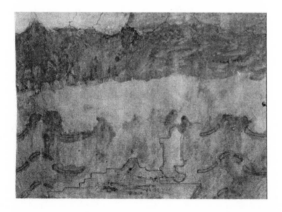

SUSAN SPLAINE

The ocean was calm sailing across it was not able to see the sunset rising in the east.
Clouds turned grey and the air went black.
The ocean became stormy when the horizon darkened.
I rowed my boat strongly and effortlessly.
I have initiative and imagination desired greater self-knowledge.

Change and progressing will keep me happy.
A transition in my life was underway.
White clouds denoted inner contentment.
In the starlit night full moon glowed.
During the day suns rays beamed down on me.
Sky and air was clear and clean.

Deterioration in the weather brought grey stormy clouds.
A rainbow was not a sign of hope.
Throughout the day sunlight disappeared behind the clouds.
At night, the moon disappeared behind the dark clouds.

DARKENED LIGHT

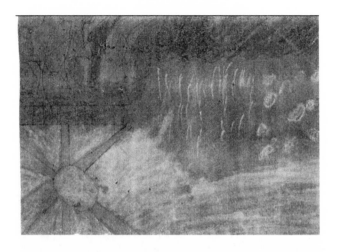

The grey skies denoted threatened misfortunes.
Stormy rain brought me feelings of pain and depression.
Hail brought me sorrow and trouble.
Ice on the ground brought me physical and emotional coldness.
A transition took place when I crossed over the bridge.
Crossing from one phase of life to another I attained peace.
Made a major decision when came to a crossroads.

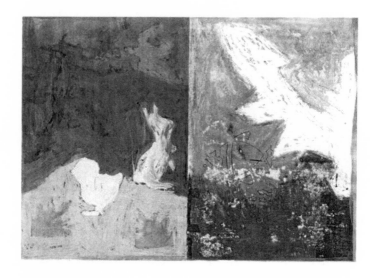

Pushed into a deep black hole did not stop me taking the journey I planned.
In a tunnel grey shadows hovered over me.
People were unfriendly I needed somebody to held a helping hand.
Suffering went on until clambered out of black hole.
This little chick learnt how to fly.
Flew like an eagle soaring in the sky.
Over the high seas, flew to a new destination like a flock of birds emigrating.
Like a hawk kept my eyes peeled on heights, targets, visions and aspirations.

DARKENED LIGHT

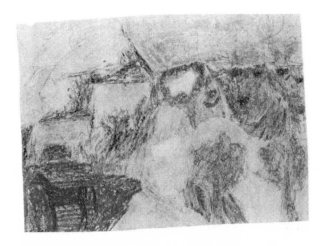

Miles out of sight could see the mountain landscape.
The shining light flickered in the distance above the mountain.
On the summit saw animals, plants and trees observed a landscape from a safe vantage point.
I made it through the isolation moments sailed the storms.
The rough, rain shine and weather conditions.

My health improved
I pushed myself to move beyond the past and into the future.
I have good intellect and creativity needed a new change in direction.
Wanted ambitions to fulfill and begin new relationships.
Pleasant landscapes blossoming trees hold out the promise of gladness and growth.

SUSAN SPLAINE

Under the misty blue skies I Searched for a new goal in life.

My life stopped moving but the world has not stopped turning.
I had gone for silver.
Always in second place in this rat race.
On the verge of a new beginning when, came to the end of the road.
At night, saw a silver star glowing in the purple sky, a full moon and the sunset.
Another dawning saw eagles soaring in the sky.

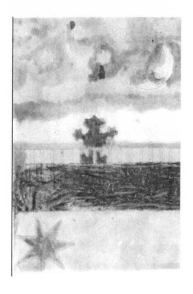

Over the ocean could see the sunset whilst standing on a bridge.
Hovering in the starlit night felt like a shadow.

DARKENED LIGHT

A star twinkling above shined brightly then fell down.
When blown in my path, the wind blew it from me.
My fallen star could not catch hold of it because was out of sight.
Spiritually I have been right beside my fallen star.
It is where I want to be giving anything and everything.
I will always care always be there.

In the far distance could see the mountain landscape getting closer.
The feeling of hope and positive ness overwhelmed me.
I wanted satisfaction and the comforts of a good life felt stronger and healthier.

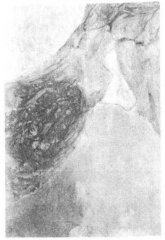

The suns rays beamed down on me from up above blue skies.

All of my bad luck stars broke so ran up hilltops reaching for my good luck stars.
I will not look back in regard to my distance.
Do not want to enter new black periods keep storm clouds at bay.

My life has not been a pleasant road. In a tunnel could not see the light. Saw red until the green light shone. Regret for vanished joys. Inside my mind, I saw images of landscapes so I drew hilltops, countryside, mountains and seascapes. On my fortune journey took one day at a time. I needed to break out of a rut could see foresee changes for the better. Dividends paid of because of my determination. Writing letters turned the tide. Took the journey I planned needed something to get my teeth into so that I could boost my confidence. Favorable times drew near because the breeze changed direction.
Gliding on ice a life of comfort over the horizon, found my satisfactory path in life.

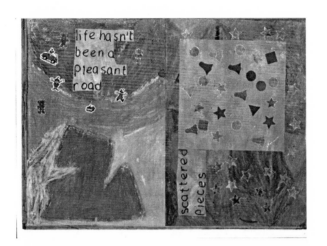

life hasn't been a pleasant road

scattered pieces

CHAPTER ONE

In September ninety-ninety-three at the age of eighteen, I was out of work. The job centre near where I lived sent me to college in Trafford where people go to do basic maths, English and job search. The staff working there saw a person within that is bursting to come out. For the first time in my life, people told me that I am bright and intelligent. On Mondays and Tuesdays, I worked in the reprographics department because I was interested in printing/photocopying. I also worked in the library when there was not anything else to do because I quickly finished a day's work.

I reached the stage in my life I realized that my personality had remained the same throughout my life. I grew up socially withdrawn, isolated, lacking in communication and social skills. At school, I was unpopular because of poor socialization. I made little or no contact with the teachers or other children. I was very unhappy, tearful, withdrawn because I felt ashamed of the funny sounds that came out of my mouth. My mum is a backward retard, has speech difficulties. I believed that I sounded like her. My mum's relatives, two sisters Freya, Griselda and brother Lenny, Great auntie June said whenever they saw me that I am like my mum, I cannot talk. My mum would comply by saying something is wrong with her. Looking back over the year's I felt cheated of my own importance and self-worth.

I am one of five children! Paddy is three years older than I am and Jasmine is two years older than I am. I am one of triplets have a sister Abbey and brother Rory. Jasmine and Rory were the too intelligent out of the five of us. They were top of the class in Math's and English. Their qualities shined through because of nurturing from grand parents, Uncle Timmy on dad's side of the family. Grandmothers on dad's side spoilt Jasmine also spoilt and nourished by Timmy those two were the favorites. Paddy and Abbey in second place as for me I was miles behind because I did not crave love or attention. I am unsure if I ever felt rejected.

At weekends and during school holidays Jasmine went to her beloved grandparent's house. Rory mostly went to his beloved uncle Timmy. We took turns going to grandparents with Jasmine. I hated going because of the close relationship she had with her grandmother. She always brought her new clothes so I had Jasmine's hand-me-downs. During the summer, holidays before going to high school relatives told me they do not want me going to their house anymore because I did not talk to them. It was not hurt because I am an outcast. Throughout my school years, I did have few friends where I securely belonged. I preferred to mix with as few people as possible. In Math's and English, I was down at the bottom of the class. My schoolwork suffered because of poor concentration. I day dreamed! I sighed a lot and bit my nails. I did not talk to anybody about my misery. How bad I am doing at school. It made me feel overwrought because relatives and teachers were disinterested in my welfare.

Paddy is the less bright and intelligent out of all of us. Last three years at primary school he went to special needs school. He did go to normal mainstream school. After leaving school, he went to college to do joinery. Every evening he came home crying and demoralized. My mum would always have his meal ready he would always throw it back at her. He could not be civil towards his mum. Every day they had arguments. They argued a lot about food because she is not a very good cook, so he took over doing the cooking. I am unsure what else they argued about because I either just left the house or cut myself off from them. I found Paddy much more annoying whenever he mellowed down and talked babyish to his mum. He does not have any special gifts or talents. He has worked as a joiner but also has been unemployed for years.

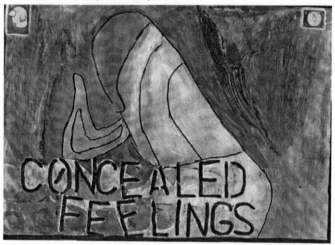

When Jasmine left school, she got a job working at all: sports. She went out in the evenings with her friend from school Scarlet, her sister and friends of theirs. Every time I went out with my school friends, Jasmine resented it. She could not bear seeing me enjoying myself. I dreaded going back home because she was always angry with me, she would interrogate me. She did not ask me where I have been because we did not have any form of a relationship. She did not ever ask me if I had a nice time. When I told, my mum I am going out Jasmine used to say tell her she cannot go. Getting dressed up and experimenting with make-up is something I have never done. She did not begrudge Abbey, Rory or Paddy going out, but why me.

In ninety-ninety, we exchanged house moved out of a four bedroom into a five bedroom. I still had to share with Abbey she is a couch potato so I could use the bedroom as a retreat, spend time on my own.

All of my life we have always had dogs. We had three pit-bull terriers Ripper, Lucy and Judy. On August 8 ninety-ninety, Lucy gave birth to ten puppies. A girl was a little runt. The other puppies put on weight, grew quicker than she did. At six week old when the puppies were eating solid food, walking around them would snap and growl at the little runt. She would sit in the corner shivering and looking tearful. Whenever I picked her up, gave her a hug that sad face broke out into a beaming smile. Nobody wanted the little runt because she was an outcast. We kept her and named her Roxy. She followed me around all over the place because we bonded together. She depended on me to love her and take care of her. She was of utmost importance to me. Caring for Roxy filled my self-esteem because she needed me; I was able to fill that need. Having her inside the house for company helped me to stop losing my sanity. She was the centre of my world. She was full of energy, full of life; she brought me so much joy and happiness because of our close relationship.

SUSAN SPLAINE

My last year at school I told the Career's Adviser I am interested in landscape work. He arranged for me to go for an interview at the Town Hall in Trafford, to get onto a training scheme with the council. I had confidence within myself that I could do landscape work for a living. Jasmine encouraged Paddy, and my mum to put me down and laugh at me. They told me that I could not do it because I am stupid. I could not live the life I wanted to live because of her controlling, dominate behaviour. I let her block me in my path from getting onto the road that just may have led to a future full of promise and happiness. I found it hard to believe in myself because I did not get any family support. Throughout my life I have always been discouraged and looked down upon as a result, my confidence is low and so is my self-esteem.

Abbey was encouraged to go to college to study childcare. She later on got a job working in an old person's home. Rory made it into employment as a plumber. The firm he worked for trained him up and paid for one-day release college fees. He traveled from place to place because he worked where plumbing jobs took him to different towns. By the time, he was seventeen he passed his driving test and had a car. I felt dissatisfied with my life and enviable of him because my life did not have any meaning to it. On my eighteenth birthday I signed on the dole my mum was so proud of me she told the next-door neighbor. She wanted half of my money. I went out to the pub across the road from the job centre. I became friendly with the barman and regulars.

Jasmine left her job working in all: sports. She got another job packing nails not far from where we lived. Where she worked needed another employee. She phoned the house and told me to go for the interview. I got the job after about two weeks she told me to leave, made the decision that I cannot do the job. I could do the work I did not do nothing wrong or make any mistakes. She spent all my life putting me down she became accustomed to doing it when it is not appropriate.

I felt as if I was on the road to nowhere because I did not have any dreams or ambitions. All I could see was misty fog. If I did not let Jasmine or Paddy be my obstacle, stop me from chasing one goal the skies would have been bluer. I let them take from me the little self-confidence I did have. If I were not such a weak person after leaving school, I would have taken my life in a different direction. When I finished college in January ninety-ninety-four, I still did not have any expectations of myself. I lived my life wishing upon a star. I waited for something to fall out off the sky that would lead to better days.

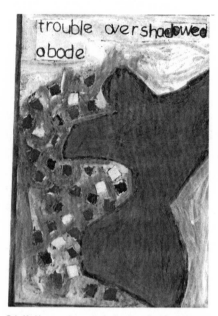

trouble overshadowed abode

Childhood memories of abuse tormented me. It became a big heaviness on my shoulders. As a child, I lived in a dream world that I belonged to a different family. It was another girl in the fantasy somebody else who could speak. We lived in Sale in a four-bedroom house. I shared with Abbey, Paddy and Rory Shared a bedroom, Jasmine had her own bedroom. We did not live on a rough council estate but we were the local tramps. My mum and dad did not take pride in where they lived so they dragged us all down to their level of trashiness. We lived in a tip, the house stunk and most of the furniture was secondhand. Nobody would ever tidy up after themselves in the kitchen it was one of the reasons why Zandra my mum shouted aloud.

DARKENED LIGHT

Ernie and Zandra's marriage was an unhappy one. They did not show or give each other love or affection, so they could not give or show it to their kids. Ernie and Zandra are not somebody to aspire too. I did not have speech difficulties because of bad genetics it was also because of upset, constantly scared because of abuse. My dad worked in a dairy he brought milk home from work. He had a routine when he arrived home. He would take off his overalls and boots he left in the kitchen. Go upstairs to wash and put his pajamas on. He was dead slow at getting ready. Every night she would shout a loud to herself, heating up his tea. She always had his tea ready. He was not the type who would come home from work and say," where's my tea". Ernie did not respond to Zandra's constant shouting saying "hurry up". "I am never going to have your tea ready ever again". "I will wait until you get in". "You're very slow". She repeated herself over, and over. Everybody sometimes would shout back at her. I reached the point I cannot take it anymore so whenever I said something Zandra would hit me. Paddy and Jasmine would tell me to shut up. I found all the shouting very distressing so I stayed in my bedroom to try escape from it all.

I was born into a family where I did not fit in or belong. The interactions between Paddy, Jasmine, Ernie, and Zandra negativity sustained between us because there was not any positively throughout my life. Jasmine encouraged Ernie to be folly with me by pulling funny faces and bend down face to face with me. He forever made up poems about me that I am from Sudan and the Turkish delight advert. He would sing to me as if he was an opera singer. I used to run out of the house all I could hear behind me were Jasmine, Paddy and my dad jumping up and down with laughter as if they triumphed over something. When I became vegetarian at the age of eleven, I had to make my own meals. Whenever Ernie came into the kitchen, I used to walk out and leave the food I am cooking in the oven. I could not bear to be in the same room as him because he would not stop pulling faces and making comments, I am a little Bamber that was Zandra's nickname. Zandra's off spring did not call her mum because all of us called her Bamber. He converted the dining room into his own lounge when I was about nine so it made it easier for me to avoid him. Whenever I passed him by in the hallway, he used to push me.

I have memories spending long periods in my bedroom. Jasmine, Paddy and Ernie behaved liked spastics and said that I am one. Whenever I was upset, they would jump up and down in my room and laugh at me. My bedroom was the room inside the house where I wanted to avoid everybody. I felt threatened by the attention I got because it was unpleasant. Zandra used to smack me and drag me about my hair just because I was upset because of their bullying. Whenever I was upset, she would say I am going to die of a broken heart. Whilst she was in the kitchen I went upstairs on purpose leaned over the banister and pushed myself over it. I remember falling to the ground; I did not break any bones. I landed on my side in front of the storage cupboard in the hallway. The kitchen door was open Zandra said, "What are you doing on the floor". I intended to hurt myself because I thought she might stop being physically abusive towards me.

Jasmine and Paddy took centre stage took on the role as head of the household. They were very bossy and terrifying. I obeyed their orders let them treat me like a house cleaner. When I said "no" I got a slap. I had to stay in my bedroom for days on end, Zandra would bring my meals upstairs to me, Paddy and Jasmine gave her permission to tell me when I can go back downstairs. I went to the shops for them; I made cups of tea and got them cold drinks whenever they wanted one.

Paddy has had a bad temper since childhood and is still arrogant and disobedient. Whenever he had one of his violent outbursts, I was always on the receiving end of it. He would try to strangle me and spit in my face. Jasmine and Paddy gave me centre of attention whenever they pulled spastic faces and called me gormless. I once brought an ice-lolly first thing in the morning Paddy forever went on about it. Jasmine and Paddy would be insolent towards me going on about the times say that I am clumsy. I do not think I did silly things to make them laugh but they found whatever it was I did funny. It is all a blur inside my mind what they used to say about me in front of me just to brighten up their life. I would be sat their and Paddy would say remember the time Sukey....and Jasmine would laugh and say something about whatever it was he was talking about. Whenever I went out with friends Jasmine, would say remember that time Sukey went out. What was so funny about that but dumb ass Paddy found it funny? I felt much more at ease and at peace with myself when Paddy and Jasmine was at their Grandparents or with Timmy and his wife Megan.

My mum had two friends Marge and Cyril who is black they lived together but had a platonic relationship. I have memories I stayed at their flat for a long period. I saw my mum whenever she came to visit. Marge and Cyril was the same old but a lot older than Zandra, I think they are at least fifteen year older than she is. Marge had a son Bevis who was in his twenties when I was just a child. Cyril was not a very good father figure to him or a role model because he is a bit of a loser. Bevis spent most of his life in and out of prison. I remember there was a bin bag in the storage cupboard full of stolen watches. Bevis and another man Ronald stayed over at the house. I do not know where Ernie was because he was not around. I have always had an image in my mind of Ronald wearing grey jeans, a grey cord jacket; he had long dark black hair.

DARKENED LIGHT

My first childhood memory I have is walking to school on a snowy, blistering cold day. My brothers and sisters walked miles in front of me. My hood kept on falling down and I did not have any gloves on so my hands were red and cold. I do not know why but I turned around and went home. I felt petrified what will Jasmine and Paddy do to me after school. My mum let me take the day of f school. She went out with Marge and left me inside the house with Ronald and Bevis. I went to bed fell a sleep under the covers in bed. I woke up without any clothes on. I remember Ronald coming into my room, sat on the bed beside me, pulled the covers off the bed. He took his clothes off then took my clothes off. He grabbed hold of my hand and made me touch him around the genial area. He also kissed me on my lips around my mouth and licked my face. On that same night, I woke up and did a wee at the end of Paddy's bed because I wanted the dog that was with him. He woke up shouting at me. Zandra came into his room shouting; Bevis came in and said that I am sleeping walking. The last time I saw Ronald is when my mum's purse went missing. I also remember the police coming round to the house looking for Bevis.

As a family, we have been on holiday three times to coastal resorts Blackpool, Butlins and Pontins. Ernie went on boating holidays on his own. He took Zandra on holiday every summer to coastal resorts. Ernie used to take us roller-skating. I did three paper rounds on Sundays, evenings and mornings because I needed the money. I brought new clothes for myself. I spent money on going out but my evening out was spoilt because I dreaded going home to Jasmine's anger I do not understand why she was so resentful and jealous. Every September we got new school uniforms. When I was twelve, I needed a new uniform before term ended because I grew out of my skirt and blouse. I brought a new one with my own money Jasmine did not believe me; she got so jealous I had to stay in my room for days on end. She gave my mum permission when I could go back downstairs.

When I was about fifteen I remember another time I had to stay in my room for days on end because somebody bleached Paddy's tracksuit bottoms in the laundry basket, I got the blame for it and a slap across the face when he shouted because he was angry he also spat in my face. I went to school, took Roxy out then my mum would bring my tea upstairs for me. Manchester United winning a football match on Sunday put him in a good mood. He had been out to watch it, Abbey taped it off the television and he watched it again. The last time Paddy beat me up I was about eighteen. Whenever I took Roxy out for a walk, she used to jump up. I did not realize that she had tipped over the bucket of water in the hallway. When I arrived home, he attacked Roxy and me because he mopped up the water. I went out to the off license brought bottles of lager and cider, drank them in the street.

I had not grown out of my childhood fears. Feeling anxious, timid I wanted my life to change but felt apprehensive about doing anything life changing, because everybody would of laughed at me and put me down. I got a lot of headaches and stomach pains. I burst into tears whenever somebody shouted at me.

On March 2 ninety-ninety-four, I woke up listening to my intuition. I had a hunch to take Roxy my pregnant Pit-bull shopping to Sale Town Centre with me. I had thoughts that something is about to happen to me. It was not a scary feeling; it felt breezy because I was glowing. At ten thirty mid morning, I took her with me just out of curiosity. I sat down on a bench a tall thin lad in his mid-twenties sat down next to me; initiated conservation with me. He asked me if my dog is a Pit-bull Terrier. I replied that she is. He wanted one of her puppies. He introduced him self as Milton. He told me also he has a Pit-bull called Dane. He was with one of his friends Deaton who was selling paintings. She felt comfortable when Milton stroked her when Deaton stroked she shivered. I arranged to meet Milton at Salford Docks on the following Saturday. Two of Milton's friends live in Salford with Deaton. Milton is originally from Sheffield, he stays at his friend's house when he is in Salford. I had problems sleeping during the nights leading to Saturday. I had butterflies in my stomach and a choking feeling in my throat.

I needed to make the effort to make new friends, have new interests if I was not to stagnate completely. I wanted good times to be ahead of me. I think being with him will put me on tip-top form. I did feel as if there was something about him he did not want me to know about when he said he goes away for a few weeks every now and then. I felt as if I needed to talk to somebody about my unhappy childhood. He might be just the person. Express my thoughts and feelings to and be surprised by his positive response, and be encouraged to go to college, study plant science, and do practical work. My horizons were still somewhat limited, it was the right time to make great

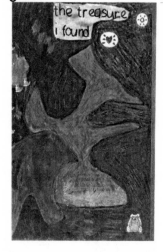

DARKENED LIGHT

I needed him to invite me to stay with him in Sheffield when there is one puppy left to be sold I want to get me out of the house I grew up in.

When I saw him waiting for me I looked at him from afar, because I was out of breath. When stood in front of him he smiled and gave me a hug. He took me by surprise because I did not expect physical affection from him. I could feel warmth from him because he is a loving person. He took me into the pub for a drink. He told me that he is a Merchant Navy Deck Officer. He had dates when he would be going away for a few weeks. I did not believe him. I think it was just a fantasy because he likes the ocean and boats. He has a barge boat called sail breeze. I managed to click with Milton. I believe in fate people meet for a reason. He took me for a veggie burger at Burger King. I went to see him everyday for the next few weeks before he went on his travels. We spent most of our time at the docks sailing his electronic boat. On his barge boat, he taught me how to steer it. As he was standing behind me, I could feel a strong emotional connection between us. I did not see much of Deaton, Kevin or Thomas his other friends. I would not talk to them. It is as if I am hiding behind a barrier. Milton was the only one who could get past it.

At home, Roxy was pleased to see me but she had a sad look on her face. I sometimes felt torn if I should stay in with her or go out with Milton. I going out was something she had to adapt to but flexibility was not in her nature. Many years living in a dream world, it felt like I fell down from the sky. I talked to him about what I would like to do for a job. He encouraged me too get onto a training scheme, maybe go to college get my life into some kind of order. Tomorrow seemed much brighter because he believed in me. I was beginning to see blue skies. I was seeking an excuse for making dramatic changes to my life. I desired to escape my present environment. I desired to break free from restrictive set routine. Milton's encouragement was enough to aid and guide me to better days. I had confidence in adapting to a new life situation.

On April 20, Roxy went into labor at about 7.00pm I comforted her in her room. She had a painful look on her face crying her heart out. The next morning at six 0'clock in the morning, the sound of a puppy crying woke me up. I went into her room she was licking her newborn puppy. That look on her face told me she wanted me to stay. Zandra was also with her. It took six hours for Roxy to give birth to all nine puppies. She was very loving and affectionate towards them. She lay still in the basket so the puppies could feed off her. She was a good mother and capable of looking after them. The last puppy left standing is going to Sheffield with Milton, Roxy and me.

I made a major decision to start a new cycle in my life. A new venture was about to happen. Milton put across his ideas about increasing my security.

I acted on my feelings and impulse. It was vital to plan and reflect on events. We found space to plan and did as little as we could to get on with it. I could sense a noticeable strength of bonds between us. We went to the cinema on Fridays. He does not drink much. It was happy circumstances me meeting Milton. Luck came my way because the quality of my life improved. I made the effort to be sociable. He was a special person in my life. Walking down the street, he smiled a lot to him self.

On April 30 my nineteenth birthday, he told me that he is a diabetic. He has to test his urine every day before breakfast and evening meal. He thought that I would not go ahead with our plans. I did not let it put pay to our relationship. It was in my own interest to get closer to him so that I could improve my life more. On Wednesday June 1, Ernie phoned the house Rory answered the phone. Somebody he worked with wanted the puppy. I decided to leave the next day because there was only one left.

On June 2, the sound of voices woke me up. Abbey came upstairs told me "it is the police they have come to take the dogs". She took Roxy and Brandi downstairs. I could not imagine my life without Roxy or Brandi. They were going to be my security when we began our new life. I could not feel the joy or excitement I felt the day before. I got myself dressed, went downstairs into the kitchen. Five male Detectives and a black woman were scattered all over the rooms downstairs. All of the doors were open. I felt in a daze. All of the dogs were in the back of a van caged up they were all barking at each other. I could not take it in she was in the van to be driven away to an unknown place.

Premier John Major ordered slaughter Pit bulls. Every dog in Britain to be put down under emergency laws. Mr. Major took action because of the horror attack on six-year-old Rucksana Khan 28 times snapping her ribs and leaving her for dead.

At five minutes past ten o'clock, the police left the house. They must be feeble minded for thinking that I could accept that had just happened, not feel any feelings about it. I went to the Off License brought a litter bottle of Wood Pecker Cider. I drank it in the park. I went to the police station because I wanted to talk to the officer who was head of the investigation he had a big grin on his face and would not tell me anything. He did not have a care in the world. The dogs committed no crime. Was not dangerous they had never harmed or caused a nuisance to anyone. Judy was pregnant. Last year she had puppies Snowy was one of her off spring we kept her because she was white. Therefore, in total five dogs, one puppy dragged from their home and incarcerated.

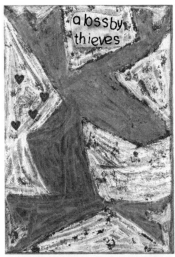

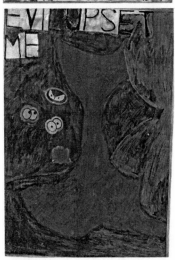

I went to Salford to give Milton the bad news. He was very disappointed because he could not have Brandi. I found it difficult talking to him because of my eyes welling up. I broke down cried in front of him. When I wanted comfort and to be held he hugged me. I kept focusing on Roxy locked up in a kennel and that sad worried look on her face. I was devastated. I let him know how much I adored her. How much she touched my life. He was very compassionate towards me. I felt like there was a big empty space in my life, pushed into a black hole.

On my first night alone without her, I felt scared inside that house. I managed to smile through my tears once I focused on how happy she had been throughout her life. I missed her so much. The police unjustly seized her from me because she did not bite anybody. I reminded myself how beautiful and precious she was to me. I had images and fantasies going round inside my mind. If I go to the police station drunk, they will give me Roxy back. They did not have a care in the world about my distress or vulnerability. I was full of rage when I over indulged with alcohol. A somewhat black period of my life had just begun. I felt resentment towards Milton because he still had his dog. I went out to pubs on my own. I felt feelings of sadness and unhappiness. I hated seeing people laughing and having a good time. I felt angry because she was gone. I had to fight back the tears because I did not want to breakdown crying in public. I was hurting inside and it showed on the outside. People asked me what the matter is. I told them about Roxy and showed them photographs. They understood that people are attached to their pets. They were sympathetic and wanted to talk to me. I had a jumbled up mind because of too many thoughts because of it and I did not think straight. I wanted to be alone. I walked the streets staring up at the sky.

Milton said he would trade places with me if he could. He cared for me a lot because we got a long. When I wanted my own way, he did not go storming off. When I was unpleasant, I did not ruin his day. I blew hot and cold with my moods. I made myself nervous the thought of driving him away. If he were not such a patient soul, I would have gotten on his nerves. He noticed a decline in my physical health. During the day, my thinking was slow because I was not sleeping much. I lost my appetite and cried constantly. Day by day black clouds rolled closer and closer towards me. I brought bottles of alcohol I stored in my bedroom. I drank before going to bed and in the morning when I got up. I got out of bed every morning walked it to Salford, visited Milton, and went to pubs on my own. We hung around the docks because I did not want to go to the cinema or bowling. I only drank a couple of drinks when Milton was with me. I did not want him to know that I was drinking a lot. Drinking in secret, I did not have to put up with him having pet talks to me that seemed like he was nagging.

I thought about when my next drink is going to be. When I wanted s drink, I had one. I drank throughout the day; I slept during the daytime. Alcohol acted as a comfort gave me strength so that I felt confident talking to people. I did not get merry when I drank too much. Summer nights men drank outside pubs. They could tell I had been crying. My eyes puffed up and red. I fell into bad habit because I talked to men who offered to buy me drinks wanting to drink drove me to put myself in risky situations. I felt empty inside I had problems all day long, staring blankly into space. Milton acknowledged that I am drinking a lot when I started turning up on his doorstep drunk. He thought that living with him was the solution to change how I felt. His attitude annoyed me and really tried my patience. I felt as if I was stuck in a rut. I did not want to move onto better things because I did not have Brandi and Roxy to take with me.

Making plans heated us both up
We could have started a fire because of the spark between us.
We both had burning desires
Everything crashed and burned.
Nothing came from the ashes because everything disappeared in a puff of smoke.
There was a time I had it all with him until it came undone.
He saw the tears I tried to hide.
He felt my heartache.
He had away to let me know he would be a shoulder to cry on.
I drifted away out of sight from him.
I felt so far apart from him.

DARKENED LIGHT

He did not feel the same loneliness, isolation, despair I felt. How could he never mind anybody else understand what I was going through? I felt edgy and nervous because I did not like life or myself seriously. I began to drink alcohol in the street instead of pubs all the time. I still carried on going to the police station drunk. I smashed bottles and cut my wrists with a carving knife. It was not a deep cut but paramedics came to put bandages on my wrist. They locked me up inside a police cell for six hours. They took the carving knife off me they let me off with a warning carrying an offensive weapon because of the circumstances why I did it.

SUSAN SPLAINE

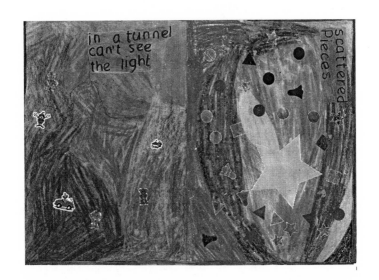

in a tunnel
can't see
the light

scattered Pieces

CHAPTER TWO

In July, I had another one of my sixth sense this time telling me to go to the job centre in Salford. I listened to my instincts because it does lead me in the right direction. A woman by the name of Maggie was recruiting people to join the job club in Salford. She asked me if I wanted to go even though I lived in Sale and was not under obligation. I decided to go to the job club, so she took my details. It is in a church not far from the fan club. Duane the job club leader traveled all the way from Yorkshire. He was a beaming, happy sort of man. He irritated me because of my obsession with unhappiness. Every day I looked in the yellow pages so I could write letters to reprographic companies because of my experience at college.

To get there I had to catch a bus into Trafford, walk it past the Docks; it was a bout half an hour walk. On my first day, I caught the bus because Maggie wanted the bus ticket because the job club refunded expenses. Every day I walked it from Sale to Salford, on Fridays got bus fares back because nobody was not aware I was not catching buses. I spent my extra money on alcohol. I used to get up at five thirty Monday to Friday just so I could be there by nine thirty. A shopkeeper served me alcohol at 8'clock in the morning. I drank it walking down the streets of Trafford and Salford.

I did not go straight home after the job club finished. I went to the cinema and bowling alley in Stockport with Milton; in Manchester I used to wonder of but in Stockport I would not because I had a fear getting lost. I think if you take the same daily route in life you might come across danger or a brief encounters. After a few days attending the job club down by the canal I walked past. I used to see the same young man who was rugged and rough round the edges. He seemed like he had problems of his own because of the glum expression on his face.

At the end of July I began to feel like I could not go to see Milton if I had not had a drink. I did not meet him at certain times because I decided to have a couple more drinks in the pub. I have always had an intense dislike for myself because of bad genetics. I have always neglected my personal appearance. I did not have a bath everyday. I did not brush my hair. I ripped holes in my jeans. I shaved sides of my hair with razors. I felt sick in the mornings and my hands shake.

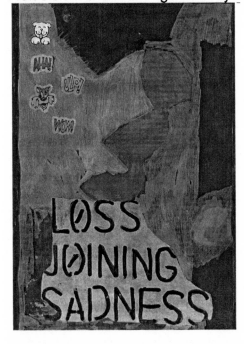

Roxy sentenced to death on September 1, I knew about it because there was an article in the local newspaper about the dogs. The government enforced Roxy locked in the kennel because she was the same breed as a dog who attacked a little girl we both had to endure not being apart of each other's world anymore. I had thoughts that I could rescue her from the prison she had been in since June. I continually found the courage to continue life without her. A thought came into my head to tell Milton to go to the police station, take an overdose of insulin in protest to get her back. I imagined he would do it for me. I went to se him before going to the job club. The back door was unlocked so I let myself in. His back to the kitchen door; the radio was on so he did not hear me come in. He was cutting up some fruit to make fruit juice he was just about to put in a food blender. I patted him on the shoulder before he had the chance to greet me; I came straight out and told him about my ideas and thoughts. All I could remember is his facial expression, his eyes wide open because he was shocked and angry. I felt a sharp knife slit my cheek it happened so fast I did not see it coming. He looked stunned and told me to leave the house. There was not anything I could do to save Roxy I felt total despair. My face was scratched and bleeding. I felt so numb it did not hurt.

At the job club, I told Duane somebody cut me with a knife. He gave me a lift to the local hospital that is just down the road. A nurse gave me a tetanus injection in my arm. A hospital social worker had a talk to me. I did not want to press charges against Milton so I told them a story behind why it happened. I cannot always distinguish what happened in reality and what has happened. Images come into mind what happened and did not happen because I am in some kind of fantasyland. Maybe I am such a good liar and cannot tell the truth. I did not show any remorse about what I said to Milton because it was as if the dark side I am seeing within took over. I blow up forcefully because I did not express inner tensions. Matters close to my heart needed a good luck at so I could find a natural release expressing inner tensions.

I knew Milton was planning to go back to Sheffield on August 27. I could see us restoring or friendship. It was important to talk to him but I was not sorry because I wanted comforting words spoken to me. I asserted myself to go and see Milton say goodbye. He forgave me for saying what I did. He put his arms around me, my eyes welling up with tears. I had a need for physical contact and warmth. He is coming back in October asked me to go and visit him

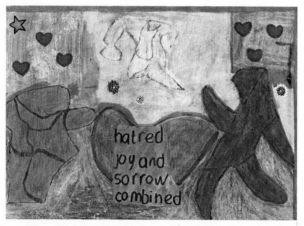

I went out looking for trouble because I think I like suffering and danger. On route to the job club, I

met up with somebody who brought me harm; just as I thought I would. The man down by the canal called Jake. He caught my attention on August 30 by smiling at me. I was drinking a bottle of mixed vodka. He asked me "what is by sorrow, my pain behind drinking in the morning". "I told him Roxy is going to die on September 1". He took the empty bottle of me and told me to phone somebody at home, I sat on the ground in the phone box he put the bottle in the bag, when Abbey answered the phone he hit me over the head with the bottle, then I hung up. He said to me if I tell the police, I will get Roxy back. I noticed he had black rings round his eyes then he wondered off. Duane phoned Salford police that was not any use because they will not tell the police near where I live. One of the men had black hair and Grey eyes just like Jake. I felt starved and empty inside because I will not get Roxy back. The two police officers drove me to the hospital where I had been for the second time. I got bored waiting so I walked it home feeling dizzy because I did not have any money.

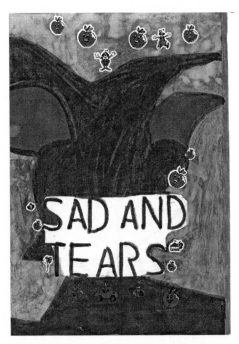

I was sick at Salford docks it was yellow. A man said to me it might be concussion, and he spoke to me I am not sure how long for. He told me that I look unwell. My eyes were black because I had not been sleeping. I had a brief encounter with a man called Alex. I felt as if I just wanted to put my arms around him because I thought we could be compatible. I could sense a spark and chemistry between us. I do not believe in love at first sight because you have to fall in love to be in love. Time stood still for me but it did not for Alex. Life was a vast wheel turning slowly because he was my dream man. I found Alex to be personable and warm; he came across as being intelligent and well educated. Alex had a negative first impression of me I had so much fog inside my head I did not want to speak. I wanted him to ask me out on a date. I drifted of into a fantasy world about him and me. I hated being alone. An idea came into my head how to get out that house. I will use Alex why I was in Salford when I do something drastic. I felt as if my life is inactive! My outlook will not always be of unhappiness and gloom because something good and exciting is going to happen. When I get out of the darkness into the light, then good luck stars will fall down from the sky.

On the morning of September 1, I went to the police station near where I lived. It was the final day of sweet, innocent dog's life. The police did not understand why I was freaking out. The reason why I felt distraught was I dreaded being all alone inside that house with people who made me the deformed freak, I am. Without Roxy my life was hell and earth. I went beyond any feeling to a grey emotional flatness. The emptiness like there is a black hole there. It was not a personal vendetta against me. Law they had to abide by ruled the police. I had a vision inside my mind protestors who opposed Pit bulls bound and joined in hostility because protestors think she was hostile. My dog did not break the law. She was not a man biter. I imagined what it must have been like for the dogs. The dogs led from their prison behind closed doors. Protecting the identity of their executioner, I do not know where the dogs were destroyed, because the location unknown to me. There is an empty space that is hallowed nothing will not fill it in, so this hole will always be there. My dog is a unique chattel. It is not possible to go out and obtain another dog like her.

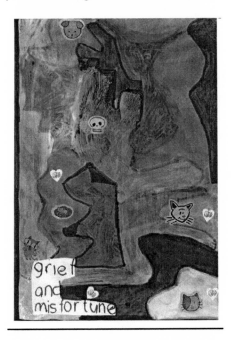

IN LOVING MEMORY

Writing about you reminds me of life's bleakest circumstances. It is the canvas of cherished memories. When seized it broke my heart. You will always be with me in my memories and thoughts. Your only mistake was to be born of a persecuted breed, slaughtered by a human hand. In death you are now eventually released soon be at home in spirit at peace with me. A small consolation to think for all that time you was sad now you are not because your soul is no longer inside your body.

The emptiness after you died was indescribable. Apart of me has gone with you. I have cried a lot in floods of tears. I miss you with every molecule of my being. I treated you right during your life. I lost you without a fight. It is hard for me to cope without you.

You were a dog of many good qualities. I was so proud that you were mine. You were special and precious to me. You gave me so much love. Timid soft, fragile were traits that made you shiver at your own shadow. You sat on my knee as if you were a small child. You followed me around the house whenever I left the room. We were always together. We spent our time going out for long walks.

FOREVER REMEMBERED

The dogs were a little group of six.
The unhappy innocent suffered.
The shock of flesh pain killed them.
I can pity I can sorrow for the pain of the dogs.
Their death was grim.
Dark clouds fell over me.
When the skies are no longer black, I will see a full moon for the first time in a long time. The black skies made the moon eclipsed. Your stars twinkle

in the night. Sparkle just like your deep brown
eyes.

All I ever wanted was Roxy.
She was the sweetest thing.
A pair of evil hands killed her.
Life is messy without her.
Time marched on.
When fallen angels fly, where do they go? She is
now my star shining down on me. No other light
will not shine brighter than ours will. Roxy was so
precious I do not want another dog because it will
not live up to her.

THE UTTERLY INOCENT

Little Roxy was the tiniest one from the start.
She was more beautiful than the other dogs.
Tiny Brandi was a dark brown colour.
She was a little beauty just like her mother.
Judy was a dark brindle colour.
You were black around your eyes.
Snowy named Snowy because she was snow
white.
She had a gift for happiness.
Ripper had a massive brindle body.
It protected his soft heart.
Lucy was the red plump one.

Their life on earth is other simply because of their
breed. Do not be curious about every spray of
light.
Sleep lazy on your pillow.

One of my earliest childhood memories is being at my Grandmothers (Zandra's mother); she had a party at her house. Family and cousins was the only people there. I saw my Grandfather on the table in front of the television. He was wearing a long brown coat just watching everybody. He did not talk to anybody it was as if he was invisible. I looked in his direction a lot because he looked sad. I wanted to say something I did not because I did not speak to people unless somebody spoke to me. I do not know how old I was when he died. I think I was at his wake after the funeral; so the vision I saw was his ghost.

I sat down by the canal with Jake drinking. I stood up to go to the job club he grabbed hold of my hand because he did not want me to go. I am not sure if he pushed me in the canal or if I stumbled into the canal. Under the water I saw my granddad wearing the same brown coat. It was as if he was in front of a tunnel, behind him I saw white or silvery colored light. He told me to go back because it is not your time. I would not turn around so he frowned at me. There and then I wanted to die. It was not my decision to make if I am going to live or die. Afterwards all I remember seeing was blue skies. Jake was bending over the bank holding my hand. I lied down out of breath. Thinking about what I saw was it real. Duane phoned the police because I was in such a nervous state I could not talk to them. Duane told me to leave the job club next time I went back because he had enough of me turning up in such a state. He even said I have upset job club members; I need to see a doctor.

I locked myself in my creations about Alex. I changed my name to Smitten Stalking because everyday I went to the docks hoping to find him. It made me feel downhearted playing game of chance. I needed to come out of my self, become somebody else then I might be able to pull somebody.

In October when Milton came back to Salford visiting friends I told him about Alex and my fantasy world. I dreamt about him all the time. Milton was very concerned about my safety and mental health. I played a dangerous game not just searching for Alex but also searching for the man who will hurt me. I had this vision once I leave home I will find that place where I will fit in and belong. On November 4 our relationship fizzled out. I lost count of how many times I said to him I will stop drinking too much I won't do it again, I mean it this time. I did not want to stop drinking. Just to keep the peace few times I did not drink when I went to visit him. He had enough of my drinking and being drunk whenever he saw me. He could not understand it was only when I was drunk I felt confident talking to people. He saw me as somebody who was unreasonable I wanted to go to the docks every day because I could not accept I will not see Alex ever again.

I stumbled, tumbled then fell. I jumped on the click wagon Milton left town, this circus also wants to leave town. I wanted to start functioning properly again make the decision to go to college next year and study horticulture. I was able to do it because I do not need support because I believe in myself; I would not have let Jasmine's and Paddy's discouragements block me in my path. I wanted to put myself together smooth over difficult times. My difficult times will not be behind me until I leave town and jump on another click wagon. This unhappy period in my life will then end.

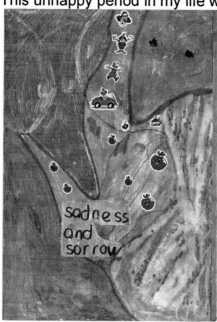

DARKENED LIGHT

At six O'clock in the evening, I was walking down Chapel Road in the dark on my way home. I did not have any money because I lost my purse. A drunken old man approached me in the street made a comment that he liked the look of me. He offered me money to have sex with him. I let him take me over the road into a car park behind a building. I let him push me into a corner pull his pants down so we could have sexual intercourse standing up. I decided that I did not want to because I was drying up; I pushed him pulled my pants up and ran across the road. I turned around he was on the other side of the road looking across at me. I went to the police station. I thought if I tell the police all about my troubles, bad times they might get me a social worker who will move me out of the house I was living in. Jamie the female officer dealing with me she was nice but we only talked about what happened. She phoned Abbey to bring me a change of clothes because I had to go to St. Mary's hospital for an examination. Rory gave Abbey a lift to the police station. Abbey went to the hospital with me. There was not any forensic evidence from the examination. I do not think nobody believed me.

A few days later a male and female Detective came over to the house, I showed them where the incident took place. It happened behind a magistrates building, then I did a statement. The police wanted to know what I was doing in Salford. I told them about Milton on that same day he went home. I told them I went to the train station with him when I did not. I spent most of the afternoon sleeping in the bed he slept in at his friend's house. I was still in a bit of a dream. I could not recall what I did when I left his house and before I got to Chapel Road.

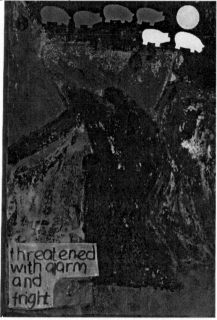

I embarked on something I did not think would fail. It did not matter where I went or what I did days did not get any brighter. I wanted lucky stars to breakthrough and shine. My mood changed easily with high and low points. I felt giddy and laughed at nothing I also cried a lot. I knew how to get out of the darkness a man had to hurt me so I could get back into the light.

DARKENED LIGHT

Snowy the new Mountain dog Paddy went to get I think from Yorkshire I hated her so much I would not stop hitting her. On he same day as Milton's birthday Taking Snowy to the police I found it was my drastic action. I wanted to come to an end of this phase in my life. The police have the authority to take unstable people to psychiatric hospital. I hoped for social workers to get involved with me. I did not want them to dismiss me because it will hinder me feeling better within myself and developing my personality. Hurting Snowy instead of myself I saw it as action to take so I could get out of that house.

I wrote a letter to explain why I took the dog to the police station.

I am scared living inside that house without Roxy. I am carrying resentment around inside me because of unhappy childhood memories that are persistent in my mind. I am full of hate, tense by bitterness and hatred towards Ernie, Zandra and her relatives. Paddy and Jasmine made my life a misery because they encouraged Ernie to pull funny faces and sing to me.

I have dug myself into a deep black hole. Now I am at rock bottom. I want an end to the misery I have been experiencing. I need help is not hard for me to admit. I want to find a way out of the darkness I am experiencing. I need to pick myself back up and face life without Roxy. I am holding onto memories of the two of us, which is why I cannot accept another dog. I just hope you will understand why I have done what I have done. I do not want anybody to visit because I do not want to see anybody. Sorrow, pain there is not a mountaintop insight. I need to get onto the road that will lead to a light of hope.

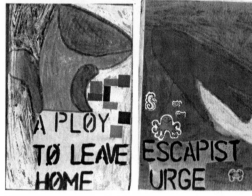

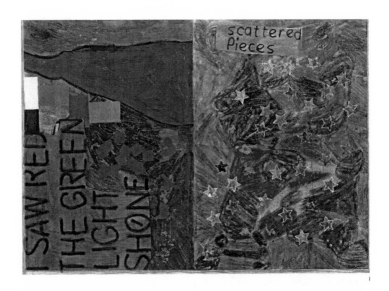

CHAPTER THREE

All day on Monday, I had another one of my sixth sense to go to Salford Docks. It was as if somebody was calling me, shouting my name. I was wearing my rose-tinted glasses because I had an image of Alex inside my head that he might be there. I did not feel scared walking the streets in the dark, because of my urge to go out to the Docks. I went food shopping during the day, treated myself to chocolate desert. I did eat my meal in my bedroom because I was engrossed in my thoughts and writing about my impending doom. I took my empty plate downstairs then took it back upstairs because my mum and Paddy were shouting at each other. I did not have desert after my meal, I walked out the house at about five O'clock in the evening, went to the tram stop in Sale.

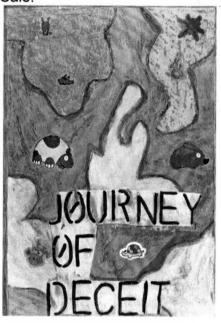

I got onto the tram to Manchester. I wondered around the fair in Piccadilly Garden's for a while. I only stayed at the fair for about ten minutes. I had small bottles of cider in my bag I drank in the street. I also had tonic water mixed with whisky. I headed towards Chapel Road. I walked past the main road through Manchester past the Arndale. I noticed the shops were still open. I carried on down the same road and came out of Bridge Street. I remember a car park on the right side of the road. There were some bus stops on the same side of the road as the car park. It was a flat car park.

At the bottom of the road, I turned left down Chapel Lane. I walked along the road for a few minutes, past some shops, a Convenient Store, Burger Bar Take Away. I did not take any notice of people I cannot remember anybody being anywhere near, me. As I carried on walking two men befriended me they noticed I looked glum. They took an interest in my personal well-being; asked me if I am lost and, where I am going. I looked at the men, but carried on walking a way from Manchester. One of them who are tall told me that his name is Ralph, the other one who is shorter than he told me his name is Lorenzo. They both had shaven hair. Ralph asked me to go for a drink with him because I needed cheering up. At this point, the two men were walking beside me. I agreed to go to the pub with them because it was how I behaved. I am not blunt, slow to trust men. Ralph held my left hand took me across the road holding my hand until we got to the pub.

We went past the Magistrates building in the car park that is where that old man wanted to have it away with me. It was as if a bolt of lightening struck twice. Lorenzo asked me if I wanted to go back to his flat. Ralph said we could go and get some pie and chips. The pub we went into had a blue door. The bar was in front of the door. I went to the bar with Ralph and Lorenzo. Ralph ordered the drinks from a woman with bleached hair that was straight with a fringe down her face. Ralph did not ask me what I wanted to drink he just ordered me half a lager. They kept on asking me if I wanted to go back to a flat and watch a video. They said we could go to another pub first. At first, I wanted to go home, but did not really want to behave as if I am naïve because I wanted them to say to me I do not want you go. Ralph did stay it is too early to go home. He told me to stay and have a good time. I said that was okay. I fell into my pattern of behaviour talking about trouble times to strangers, and showing photographs of Roxy. I gave the impression there is bad blood between the police and I; I will not report you if an attack happens. When we drank, our drinks left the pub to go to another pub across the main road.

The pub had a dark burgundy colored door. As we went through the door, we went through another door to get to the bar. The bar facing us as we went into the room I sat down. Ralph asked me what I wanted to drink. I told him Martini and Coke. Both men went to the bar. I sat and watched the news on television whilst those two get the drinks. Ralph and Lorenzo spoke to some people in the pub. Ralph came over and sat next to me. Lorenzo carried on talking to the people in the pub. The barman shouted taxi. Ralph got in front next to the driver. I sat in the back with Lorenzo. Ralph spoke to the driver but Lorenzo and I did not say anything.

DARKENED LIGHT

It was about a four-minute drive to get to the other pub. I did not recognize the area so I am not sure where I went. The pub is on a side road. There are some terraced houses adjoining to it. There were windows on both sided of the pub door. We walked straight ahead then left to the bar. Ralph asked me what I wanted to drink. I told him whisky with lemonade.   Ralph put his arms around my neck and shoulders. He asked me again to go back to the flat. He told me if I went to the flat with him, he would give me £6 for taxi fare to get home. I thought he was being friendly so I agreed to go back to the flat with him. Ralph phoned another taxi then we left the pub. Ralph sat in the front again; I sat in the back with Lorenzo. I had rips in my jeans Lorenzo touched my thigh whilst we were going to the flat. I told him to stop it he moved his hands. Those two could not see my inner self who is dark as a result could not see the wood for the trees. A couple minutes later, the taxi stopped in a small car park.

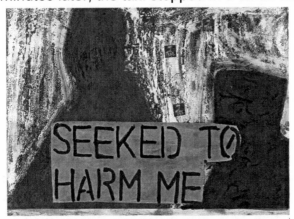

We all got out of the taxi, walked round a corner of a block of flats. The doors were glass and had big metallic handles. Lorenzo got to the door first opened it with a key. He walked in followed by Ralph and me holding hands. Lorenzo pressed the button on the lift for it to come down. It was empty when we went into the lift. Ralph let go off my hand in the lift. The lift stopped on the second floor. We turned right and went to the front door of the flat. The doors were all peach colored. The number on the door is 45. Lorenzo opened the door there were two locks for him to open with two separate keys. We all went into the flat. First, we went into the hallway. The lounge was on the left side. The kitchen was facing the living room. The bathroom was next to the kitchen. There was a bedroom on each side of the living room.

We all went into the living room I sat on the couch. Lorenzo put the television on then made some drinks vodka and lemonade. Ralph sat next to me on the couch. I did have thoughts going round inside my head "you are going to rape me are you not". There was one chair in the lounge and a wall cabinet. There were some photographs of children on the cabinet. The drinks were also in the cabinet. There was also a coffee table in the room. The carpet was multi colored, and the couch and chair were grey, brown and stripy. There was not a shade on the light. Coronation Street was on the television. Lorenzo and Ralph were whispering to each other. Lorenzo had sat down on the sofa next to Ralph. Ralph had his arm around me. He leaned over and put my drink on the table with his other arm.

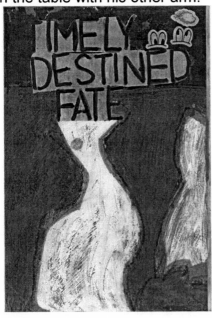

Ralph took off my jumper and Lorenzo took off my boots. Ralph said, "It is just a bit of fun". I behaved as if I was frightened "I want to go home". He told me I am not going home until tomorrow because I am staying the night. Ralph undid my jeans and pulled them down. I sat on the edge of the couch trying to pull them back up because I do not have the greatest body. Taking all of my clothes off it happened so fast. Lorenzo threw my jeans over to the other end of the room. Lorenzo had taken his clothes off as well. Lorenzo sat on the couch next to me. Ralph was kneeling on the floor in front of me. Ralph penis was not hard. He was biting my breasts and pulling them. Then he started licking my legs on the inside of the top of my legs. Lorenzo was touching my back, neck and hair. Somehow, I ended up on the floor. I think Ralph pushed me or they both did. I was lying on my back Ralph got on top of me. I could feel his penis against me it felt big and hard. I was very tense he kept on saying relax and enjoy it. Lorenzo was watching us. He was kneeling down on the floor behind my head. Ralph kissed me on the face, lips and stomach. I wriggled about trying to push him away, but he kept on doing it. He also kept on trying to push his penis inside me he had pulled my legs open. He kept them open because of his body weight. I was not moist so he could not penetrate me.

Ralph said I should have a bath to help me relax. Lorenzo went to the bathroom to run some water in the bath. Ralph got up took hold of my hand and led me to the bathroom. It was if he was dragging me behind him. I got into the bath and Ralph washed me. Lorenzo was not in the bathroom. When I got out the bath, Ralph put a towel round me and patted me dry. Ralph took me to the bedroom; Lorenzo was already in there lying down on the bed. There was just a mattress on the bed. The sheets and quilt were on the floor. I felt tired out and just wanted to relax. We all lay down in the same bed. I was in the middle of those two. After a while, Ralph knelt down in front of my face and put his penis inside my mouth. It was still hard. Lorenzo was touching my legs and vagina. He was also masturbating me.

They both changed places and Lorenzo put his penis into my mouth. Ralph lay down next to me. He kissed me on my neck, sucked my breast and touching me all over. Lorenzo licked the inside of my vagina. They were both sexually stimulated. The erectile tissues filled with blood making their penis erect and firm. During sexual intercourse, Ralph has inserted his penis into my vagina; he did not stimulate my sex organs so he could not move his penis back and forth because I was not sexually stimulated it caused him not to have rhythmic contractions. Ralph got out of bed hit me with a towel saying I am naughty because I was tense. He left the bedroom to go and get some chips. He went into the living room to get dressed. I could not find my knickers so I just put my jeans on. Lorenzo stayed in the bedroom. I was looking for my jumper when Lorenzo left. I found my jumper and put it on.

Lorenzo came into the living room took my clothes off again. I told him to stop it because I did want to go home. He led me back into the bedroom. He had my clothes in his arms. He put my clothes onto the floor then pushed me onto the bed. I tried to get up but he would not let me. He tied my hands to a bed board with a tie. Then he tied my other hand to the opposite side of the bed with a tie. I struggled to set myself free. I could not because they tied to tight. He tied my legs to the legs at the bottom of the bed with some more ties. He got on top of me and kissed me on my face. I was very unresponsive because abuse and nobody loving me made me repressive. He kept on trying to put his penis inside me. It was physically painful when he inserted it. I told him that I could feel something dripping from my vagina. I was bleeding from my vagina. Lorenzo untied me and said I could go. He ran the water for me so I could have another bath. I could see that he had blood on his penis. Whilst I washed myself in the bath, Lorenzo wiped the blood from his penis using a towel and water from the sink. He gave me a stripy colored towel. I dried myself in the bedroom then got dressed. He then told me I could stay because it was eleven 0'clock at night.

I phoned up Abbey told her I am not coming home tonight. Lorenzo spoke to her on the phone just to confirm it. He made me a cup of coffee for me then changed his mind about sleeping in the spare room. He left the flat with me down the stairs to take me to a taxi office. We could not find one so he ran off. Left me in the street near to where the job club is. I lied down in some bushes because I planned to spend the night there. At some point during the night I think I wanted to go to the police station which was not so far away instead, I went into Manchester where a lady tramp approached me because I had blood dripping from me I told her what had happened to me. I decided to wait until the morning to make my report so I went back into the bushes.

DARKENED LIGHT

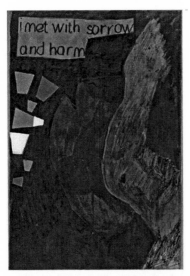

I did not find it a trauma because dirty linen will come out in the wash. Skeletons in the closet will come out. I threatened myself with alarm and fright because of sorrow and sadness. I subjected myself to an ordeal on that night. Sexual activity was vaginal, penetration and oral. Pain of mind and grief is how I found myself suffering weary. It came in mental pain, suffering helplessly because I humiliated myself. Those two were not ashamed did not blush because they were not sexually satisfied.

Early next morning at seven o'clock in the morning, I got up and made my way to the police station. There was blood on my inner thigh during the night I bleed heavily. I sat outside the police station for about twenty minutes drinking a bottle of cider I had in my bag. I needed alcohol in my system to give me strength to report wrongdoing.

I told a stern looking old woman on the reception that two men raped me. She asked me for my phone number, name and address, she phoned up my house told somebody to come and take me home. I told her two men dragged me into a car because I presumed the police were not going to do anything about it. I felt confused because of the old crone.

Detective Ivan Faith came out to the reception he sounded irrigated when he asked me if I have been drinking all night, is that it. "You have been here before have you not"? He took me into a tiny room. He put a plastic sheet onto a chair so I would not get blood on it. A woman police constable sat in the room with me reading a magazine. She did not ask me any questions so I did not talk to her. I was waiting for somebody to come and take me home. After a short while, Ivan came back into the room saying has she said anything yet. She told him that she could not get anything out of me. Ivan left the room I felt obliged to tell her what happened the night before. She then put her magazine down, sat much closer to me and wrote down notes.

Ivan came back into the room has she told you anything yet. I was being much more forthcoming about three in the bed romp. Will and graces drove them to have a sex party. Ivan sat with me for about twenty minutes I told him more about the night before. Two men stripped me off my clothes one watched the action whilst the other one had a go molesting me; then the other had a go and the other one watched. I drank cider out of water tonic bottles. I did not have labels on the bottle so I told Ivan it is pineapple juice. He looked in my bag and poured my bottles down the sink. That woman constable had to go to court so another constable sat with me.

Ivan drove us to St. Mary's Hospital; he also took the blooded sheet with him for me to sit on the backseat of the car. A female doctor examined me. A counselor helped her with the medical examination. A photographer took photographs of bruises on my chest and a handprint on my backside. Ivan and the woman constable waited for me until I had a shower. Traumatized by rape I was not because it was not an ordeal. Two perverts I did not think it would happen thrown into my path by the chances and changes of life it was very harmful indeed. My main need is more self-confidence and self-worth. Feeling down in the dumps, I found the day something of a drag, stop and go feel about the day. I went through with Ivan what I had already told him. I had an image of Burger King inside my mind because I think it was near the flats.

Ivan drove me to Salford Shopping Centre to see if I could locate the flat, but I could not. When Ivan drove me home at five thirty in the evening, he told my mum that I had a bad night. The mood at home was not delirious happy. I bottled up my bitterness I felt towards the people I lived with because they drove me to the brink of despair. If only everybody would stop shouting every day. Ernie still pulled funny faces at me even though Jasmine is no longer there to encourage him. I felt downhearted because I had to make a fool of myself because it is only my way out to get a way from everybody.

Max Clifton was the Detective who led the investigation. On November 23 I did my statement with Beatrice she came round to my house picked me up with Frederick who drove me to St. Mary's Hospital where I did my statement. They decided it would be much more comfortable me doing it there as opposed to a police station. I did the statement on my own with Beatrice Frederick went somewhere and Max picked us up. I managed to express myself to her about what happened in graphic detail, what they did to me. I did not get tearful even though thoughts were bad not good. Granted a wish was just inside my head but I could see my life will lead to brighter days instead of being grey and unexciting. Themselves unmoved with hands by evil stained. The thing they did most was to show temptation was not slow. They had the power to hurt me. Max did not come into the house to tell anybody what had happened when he drove me home. I think he was in a hurry to get home to watch Manchester United.

I did not tell anybody what had happened. It was not hard for me to accept I committed in sin and played the role of a victim. Moments came in my life when there was not anything to do but suffer. Those two created out of fantasy inside my head and put into action. Ninety-four comes across as being an unlucky year but under the circumstances, it was not. From what seems bad luck I can gain and rebuild my life back up on solid foundations? I want to move into a much cheerful atmosphere.

On November 27, Frederick phoned to inform me that he has some good news, he picked me up drove me to the police station just to tell me him and Max has arrested Ralph and Lorenzo The second pub we went into the police did there investigation there. Ralph and Lorenzo were regulars in the pub so they were well known. When the police went into the pub to do, their investigations Max and Frederick explained on Monday the girl with Lorenzo and Ralph they raped her in a flat. People who were associated with Ralph and Lorenzo acknowledged it was wrong what they did to me, so they gave the police their address and told the police their surnames. The flat is Lorenzo's mothers it was empty because she was on holiday. Lorenzo spoke to the police but Ralph did not. When Frederick drove me home, he told my Zandra and Ernie what had happened. Paddy said he is not bothered it was what I expected of him because he is not a brother to me. Everybody will always be unsupportive so people will have to cope on their own during their darkest hour. Why does my life have to be full off sorrow? Do I mean to hurt myself but I do not cry about it.

On December 5, Beatrice drove me to Middleton police station because I had to identify Ralph. Abbey also came because she had to do a statement with Max because she spoke to Lorenzo by phone. The property owner and his wife from the second pub also came to identify Ralph. He was number four. He looked liked such a lost soul.

I did not have any counseling because I am a freak. I felt rejected and placed out in the cold because I did not have anybody to listen to my thoughts about hell on earth. To help me through my struggles I thought about if Milton were, still apart of my life he would give me love and affection because he was not prejudice against me. I was aching with sickness I wanted Milton to say I care. On January 6, Milton sent me a postcard from Spain. He wrote a message at the back come visit me in Salford next month. I did not go because I felt like I could not face him. I cut back on outgoings. I isolated myself in my own confinement from the outside world. I enjoyed being on the fun side of life with Milton but it was only a short-lived relationship.

DARKENED LIGHT

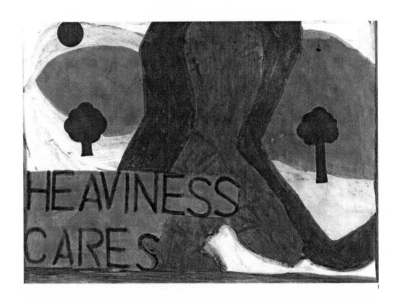

In the midst of despair, I wrote letters to Crown Prosecution. I felt very unsettled and full of inner turmoil I wanted to express my feelings to somebody. I dragged myself down because not every day was any different from the rest. I let experiences of this last year occupier my thoughts. I could not relax at night. My face burnt up. I got pins and needles in my legs and arms. I had butterflies and a sickening heaviness in the pit of my stomach. I went to the toilet a lot to pass urine. I was up most of the night going to the toilet. I got many physical symptoms I think because of stress and memories from my childhood. I am not sure who made me appointment at Victim Support in Sale the woman who dealt with me gave me a form to fill in to apply for compensation. I could get unto ten thousand pounds. It was the one and only time I saw her. I wanted help and understanding because it was difficult for me to maintain a sense of balance with my moods.

I still drank a lot because my life was humdrum and boring. I spent long periods in my bedroom during the evening and throughout the day. I moved into the bedroom Rory slept in, Jasmine left home so he moved into her bedroom. All I seemed to do every day was writing. I did not just write for my first three chapters but for other chapters I will do. Most of this book is about my thinking and thoughts. Sometimes it seems like it is not me thinking but my inner self so it takes over. My life has not been a pleasant road over the years I have been in a rut for years. I let men trample over me because thoughts of deceit occupied my thoughts. Was I their lucky number? I had an image in my mind seeing myself on top of a cliff looking down from a great height, and looking ahead to new horizons because I did not have a sense of direction. I did not have any ambitions. Hopes or dreams to come true in the immediate future. I was on the road to nowhere. When the misty fog eradicates then the end will be insight begin again on a new open road. I hoped I would find a great deal of common ground and setbacks bring me new hope. I waited for something good and interesting to happen. I hoped that the wind of change would blow me in the direction where the black cloud will drift from over my head. I am not afraid of changes. When

I get into a better frame of mind, I will better myself.

In May 1995, I found my mum's medication in the kitchen cupboard she took for headaches and blood pressure. She did not take her prescribed medication. At night, I took two with whisky and lemonade. If I got up early, I took two more with alcoholic drinks. I stored bottles in my bedroom. The tablets made me feel dreary and tired. I wanted to sleep all the time because I was in a lazy frame of mind. My pupils were dilated, contracted and my eyes welling up with tears.

I had dreams about family life and cozy domestic bliss. My husband was not Alex he was Stone. He also did not look like Alex. Stone was rugged, mean and moody looking, rough round the edges. He had brown hair and brown eyes very tall just like that; man is from the x files. I do not know his name I saw a clip of an episode flicking through the channels. I had a baby boy called Storm. He looked like his dad. If my dream was true, I think I would be working as a horticulturist. I will not ever meet anybody who is my soul mate. A difficulty I have will stand in my way of ever having relationships. I come across being shy but I am not, I am just ashamed to talk that is why I stay silent. There are lonely people in the world because there is not somebody out there for everybody. Getting onto the road to happiness will not be because I have a boyfriend. Men who are warm and loving and make me feel secure. I would like to have a man who is loving and affectionate. I think negative the chance will not come to me to be responsive to love.

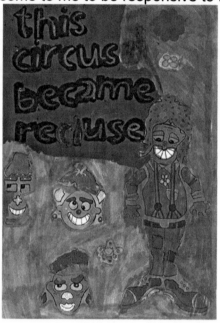

In June, Jasmine came round to the house I was in bed at 6.30pm; Abbey came upstairs to get me out of bed. Jasmine noticed that I did not look a picture of health. She told her old school friend Scarlet so she got involved in my troubled life. I took a different direction to cope with my emotional state and dealt with it. She arranged for me to claim sickness benefits because I was still on the dole and having restart interviews at the job centre. Scarlet took me to the doctors to get a sick note. He wrote depression. I also took medication for my psychosomatic symptoms going to the toilet a lot. My doctor also arranged fro me to se a psychiatrist who should get me social workers. I always thought psychiatrists only see people with mental illness and out patients. They are not therapists; do not take a person on a journey of self-discovery to find their way back to how they used to be before they became unwell. During assessments when a person is a patient in hospital a psychiatrist might delve into a patients past and childhood. Scarlet took me to a rape crisis centre in Manchester I could not talk to the counselor during the session. I think it was because all I could see inside my head was grey clouds what happened on that night seemed like such a blur.

For six weeks every week Scarlet came with me to have counseling at AA in Sale; I did talk to her but did not always make my self clearly understood. I will not ever be able to have a proper conversation if people. I am unsure if it is because I am not confident or if I do sound like my mum. If I do have her speech difficulties, then why am I not backward and have the mental age of a child. I still carried on drinking because I hate my mum for what she is. I drank before I went to counseling sessions even though I was anti-depressants. I did not care if mixing alcohol and tablets would make me ill. I swallowed down my medication with alcohol. All the time I felt like I want to drink. I could not fight my cravings because they were much stronger than I was. I did not want to give up or say good-bye until this stage of my life is over. I only have one failing but because of it, I will always hate myself.

On Tuesday 26 September Jake sent me a note saying he is going to kill him self. It felt like the right timing to take an overdose so Social Workers will get involved with me. I was feeling fed up every day so I wanted things to get moving and make some changes. I used Jake's note as the reason why I did it. I brought a bottle of cider and swallowed down about six anti-depressants and about three of my mum's tablets. As I was, making my way to the local hospital the police saw what I was doing and phoned an ambulance. At Trafford Hospital I had pulse and heart rate tested on a monitor. Jasmine came to see me with her fiancé (I have forgotten his name). We waited six hours to see a psychiatrist. I did not get what I wanted to go into the psychiatric hospital that is on the same hospital grounds.

All I could talk about was my resentment towards the police because of what happened with Roxy. We talked about Jake where we met, the doctor wanted to know how he knew where I lived. I must have given it to him. The doctor took his note of me and did not give it back. I felt more despair because all I want is to get away from Paddy' and Zandra is constant shouting. I had belief in myself I will find away out. Jasmine and her fiancé drove me home. I went straight to my room. Zandra shouted aloud why she did it. Abbey and Jasmine shouted back why you think.

DARKENED LIGHT

My unsupportive family did not give me any comfort because it was not comfort what I wanted. To be loved I do not have a desperate need for it. I want an end to my misery cover up the black hole I am in so I would not fall back in to it once I gotten out. I filled my physical hollowness with alcohol. I did not get headaches because of hangovers.

In October, I began to hear voices. Do it, kill you. On October 11, I woke up thinking I am going to take another overdose. The night before I packed my bag with diaries, compact disc, personal stereo, books to read, toothbrush and tooth paste. I left the house with a bottle of cider, my mum's medication. Walking down the street heading for the local hospital, I swallowed the medication down with alcohol. I told the receptionist woman that I have taken an overdose. A doctor who spoke to me phoned Trafford Hospital to let them know because he made a referral for me taken to Trafford Hospital. On my way to the ambulance I had a black out in the car park. I was unconscious for about five hours. I woke up vomiting and with monitors connected to me; male nurse was looking into my eyes with a torch. He asked me for my phone number so he could inform my family where I am. When he came back to my bedside, he wrapped me up warm underneath three blankets because it gets cold in the corridors.

I stayed on a ward with women of all different ages most of them were elderly. Four days, I stayed on the ward a psychiatrist who I had not seen before (because I have seen two at Trafford Previously) came to talk to me. I talked to him about feeling discarded I needed some kind of therapy but nobody do not seem to want to help me. Life has not been treating me well. My mum and Scarlet came to see me. Jasmine phoned to ask me why I am in hospital. I told her mentally I am sick. The psychiatrist referred me to the psychiatric hospital. I accomplished my mission because I am persistent. My mum told me social workers have written to my house because they wanted to come and see me at home. If they are not bad apples, they will move me to a different town.

I was not very good at expressing myself to doctors or nurses who spoke to me. I expressed my feelings by pulling a sad face and crying in my room. Scarlet and family members came to se me. Paddy, Rory, and Ernie did not. I smiled or laughed when I described hostile feelings. Inside I cried constantly but could not show how much I was hurting or show my pain the real reason why I did what I did. I was inside hospital for two weeks. I spent my time in my room reading and writing. Withdrawn from people and staying within me, it felt safe. The external world was of secondary importance because of my fantasy life not about Alex anymore but Stone and Storm. I watched television in the lounge. I brought alcoholic drinks from the local convenient store. I did speak to an elderly woman, another young woman and an Asian lad. I agreed with doctors that social workers are the ones to get involved in my dead-end life.

I do not want to see a psychiatrist as an outpatient for the long term because I do not suffer from mental illness. During sessions doctor and patient talk about how they feel due to their illness. Talk about their feelings and behaviour. Doctors and patients talk about if they have felt well or unwell. Across the road from Home from Home, which is a day centre for people with mental health problems, is a practice where my consultant psychiatrist goes. I might see her once or twice as an outpatient. It was hard for me to accept that doctors were bothered about me because I hate myself because I have my mum's bad genetics that makes me sound like her. I think there is a stigma against me; doctors are not living without prejudice. I packed my bags and discharged myself. My key worker Millie phoned me at home I told her I feel okay when I was not. My mum went to the hospital when I was not there.

SUSAN SPLAINE

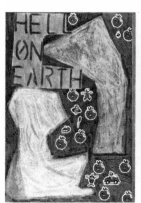 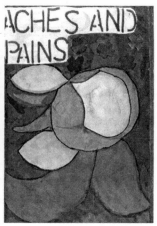

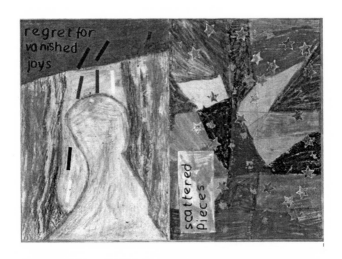

CHAPTER FOUR

Hilda Barrie and Benjamin Leighton were the two mental health social workers appointed to come and see me. They came round to the house to talk about what I need help with. I had been suffering in silence because I did not have a helping hand. I spent too much time on my own. I drifted into a negative mood so life seemed to be against me. Hilda and Benjamin found my naivety and innocence touching. It seemed like I was living life in pain and discomfort because of disappointments, disturbances and upsetting experiences. My mind was not relaxed because of too many thoughts about my loss childhood; all I want is to get a way from Paddy, Ernie and Zandra. I did not feel at peace within myself

89

because I was stuck inside a very deep rut. I was not able to solve difficult times. My life had gotten to be a bit too much it appeared my entire existence was about the state of my health because I felt as if I was on the verge of a breakdown. I found getting headaches and sore throats a lot too much to cope with. I need to mature and grow so that I can find my personality. I do not know how to describe myself because I do not know what my true nature is.

I have not been able to form stable relationships because of feelings of inadequacy. I needed to seek help to understand why I am so inferior about speaking. I feel ashamed of the funny sounds that came out of my mouth. The only reason why I feel inadequate is my mum's bad genetics inside my head I hear her loud horrible voice, but what I hear I do not know if the same sounds come out of my mouth. Since childhood, people have judged me and compared me to a mental retard. I do not think people think to themselves she sounds like her mum; nobody cannot begin to understand or imagine what it is like having a mum like her. I have always been unhappy because of my problems feeling uneasy, uncomfortable talking to people. I want guidance to manage myself more effectively if I get away from Zandra, I might sound different and speak in a different accent.

I do not feel as if I have wasted time on reflection because I have written about my reflective thoughts. Hilda and Benjamin found it difficult communicating with me because of my state of mind because I am not confident speaking to people. I traveled down the road that led to desperation and isolation because I kept them both at arms length I missed out what was going on under my nose. I found it hard to accept they will not judge me because nobody as ever had been bothered about a spastic like me.

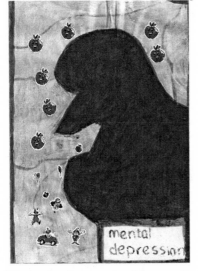

They took me to Home from Home that is near Sale Town Centre. It is a day centre for people with mental health problems. Upstairs people stay in the residential area when they feel unwell. There are eight bed-sits, bathrooms, toilets, television lounge; a member of staff sleeps over every night. I overheard a man at the day centre talking about the X Files, I would of liked to watch it just to glare at the leading actor and just be mesmerized by him, but I could not watch it because Paddy decides what to watch on television. I am sure Stone came into my dreams because I had a longing to watch the X Files, because there are facial similarities between them.

New faces and places will no doubt give me a different slant on life. People in authority looked very kindly on me. Problems had been plaguing me for sometime. Repressive anger needs unblocking within me because of the anger I feel about Ernie, Paddy and Jasmine bullying me. I wanted to breakdown and cry but the tears would not come. Hilda, Benjamin and support workers from Home and Home were being honest with me, and wanted to help to ease the pressure I had been enduring. My secret fears seem to indicate the time came to let down my defenses.

The more I am ready to give out to people the more they will be responsive to me. A change must come and new beginnings or life will stagnate. Whatever they offer I should take it because I never know whether the chance might come again. I am very persistent and apply passive resistance. Hilda and Benjamin will budge but will not have to bribe me to move out of that mad house, because getting out of there is what I want. I went to the woman's group I did not talk to anybody because I was not interested in anybody's problems or troubles. I am not a good listening I do not know what to say to people because I am inarticulate. The chances were that eventually the group leaders would have caved in on me. Action, thoughts and longings is what life is all about.

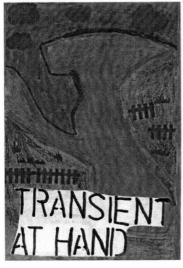

I thought about my impending court trial: The judge, Jury, Barristers will see me as a deformed freak. The rape did not affect me but it does have an affect on me judged wrongly that I do not have any feelings. I do not have the communication skills to communicate what I think and feel about what happened. My communication problems do also centre on my ability to absorb and understand other people's point of view. It took fourteen months for my double rape trial to go to court. In court plots were hatched against me on that night. I also plotted and schemed. Scarlet proved to be a source of support. Abbey also had to go because she spoke to Lorenzo on the phone on the night. I made a start dealing with matters that have been hanging around for sometime. I let Ralph and Lorenzo make my life a misery just so I could find new ground. I was down in the dumps, made a fool of my self-searching for that place where I fit in and belong. If only the police, Lorenzo and Ralph knew my motives. It might take time for those to live it down when my secret becomes public because I took them for a ride.

Barristers did not read out my statement in court. The jury did not know what happened on that night because nobody told them because Barristers did not put across details to them. The Barristers did not show forensic evidence in court. Barristers used letters I wrote to crown prosecution as evidence in court. I did not hold back on my thoughts and feelings in writing because I went through rough patches on my own. The man in my dreams Stone I saw him inside my head. He was laughing, sneering at me. It was difficult for the jury, barristers and judge to understand because I was nervous and stammered. I had a choking feeling in my throat and a headache. I felt as if that big black cloud had returned. I was reserved and reticent because I did not matter. My stresses, strains and struggles were all that mattered. A rape trial was not about a rape. Ralph and Lorenzo showed me no fear. They were penitent. The defense barrister behaved forcefully because he was domineering. Those two were the choosers. I suffered in pitiable suffering. I can only accept that it happened. What is the ultimate purpose and meaning of it? I do not understand if there is an outside force did fate and destiny meet us up at the pick up point. I will not ever know because it is lives mysteries.

Two men sat in pairs were awed in spite of themselves. Defense barristers guided them: From his lips, heart-rending cry in all sorrowful history of humanity, "she trapped these two men, they should go free". He startled me! That he so meek and yet so strong should have had that agonized cry wrung from him. It is that fundamental problem which he did not find answered. That is why he gave his power to believe in Ralph and Lorenzo. It is proved and demonstrated by the fact that the wrath of him with all ungodliness, unrighteousness, upon imprisonment because those two were not meant to go to prison because my dark side took over during my desperation. He went to all the lengths against evil, because of the length he went to a verdict was not reached. The Barrister rescuing them from evil is a rescue from themselves, from their false selves. It was not painful for me because my actions were also evil. The rape then is not just a tragic and pathetic incident, a misunderstanding, a perversity of comparatively two men.

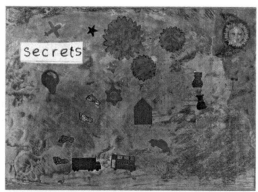

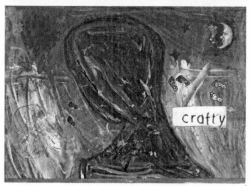

Beyond all this, everything that has happened there is much more agonizing moral problem which life presents unceasingly. In spite of all my faults, in spite of all my sins there is not apart of me who has no aspirations for good. I saw good triumph because I was on the verge of leaving home. My cry was not just that it is over. It was a shout of triumph and accomplishment. I thought that I overcame the world. It was possible through the grossly exaggerated lips of their defense Barrister. Nobody heard the proof because all that matters were letters I wrote to the Crown

Prosecution. I wrote them because I had a compulsion to write letters not to them but also to allsorts of organizations; I did not understand why letters were relevant to the case. It was a struggle of humiliation, before victory. I think my suffering would have meaning and worth if I get away from my trashy family; frustration triggered me to humiliate those two. Hurting myself the way I did people who have been sexually abused find sex attacks traumatic but I did not.. Lose their pride and dignity, weakness, the indignities of all kinds suffering is enduring strongly humanly.

In life, I have had my difficulties, distresses and sorrows; I do not understand why I feel joy because I do not have anything to feel joyful about because I do not have anything in my life. I am inside a black hole. There seem to come so much by chance, so little merited that life for me is not an easy thing at all. It is not only that it has brought great and crushing sorrows, pains and anxieties. In the process of life itself, there is hardness, a stress and straining after something beyond itself that grinds and hardens us against our own wills. Does it have to be this way? Does anybody care?

I compare the troubles I underwent in a cause of a year. I took the burden appointed for each day. I did not choose to carry my troubles by carrying yesterday's stick over again today, adding tomorrows burden to my load before I am required to bear it. I went down the same roads and the same streets on the prowl. I gave them signals to attack me. Everyday life seemed unimportant in comparison to finding a way out of that house and my awful experience. The pain of loss childhood is real just like putting my self in a position where two men will attack me is real. I will not forget but the memory does not hurt.

After two days, my court trial discharged because I am a spastic and a freak not because there was not enough evidence or proof. Why was there a court trial if Ralph and Lorenzo were not going on trial? It was silenced there side of the story. I was the only witness during the trial. There was not anybody on my side. That defense Barrister believes in flying pigs because he believes a freak like me gave Ralph and Lorenzo the wrong impression. He said something as I trapped them because of the police and the dogs. He was not aware of my vulnerability because I did not tell anybody my secret. I think the media will laugh at Ralph and Lorenzo during the midst of controversy when my secret is public knowledge. Those two left court standing tall with their pride intact. I did not have any rights just wrongs. They went down the road where the sun is lighting up the sky. I went down the road where it has stopped raining because the black clouds were drifting.

DARKENED LIGHT

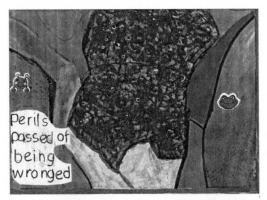

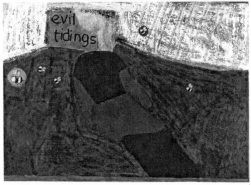

SUSAN SPLAINE

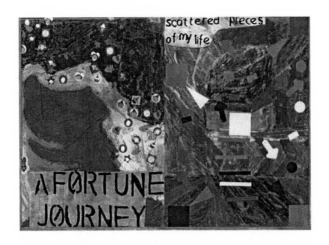

CHAPTER FIVE

On January, I8th social workers moved me into Home from Home where I stayed for 8 weeks. Without confidence, I will not go far. Confidence is static keeps a person together. If my circumstances were different, I would be different. If only I was somebody else and had their chances. If this, that and the other might be all would be well with me. I should never picture myself under any circumstances in which I am not. Never compare myself with that of another. Never allow myself to dwell on the wish that this, that had been or were otherwise it was. I began to trade in things that do not exist. I lose my peace of heart because I have begun to trade something that is unrealistic. There is no joy in things that do not exist.

SUSAN SPLAINE

I locked myself away in my own confinement within myself. I have powers of imagination. I combine a vivid active imagination **with** a creative mind. It comes natural to me cutting myself off from the outside world. News that I am getting compensation came my way. I can now pay my catalogue debts.

My Social Workers have contacts at a psychiatric home **in** Blackburn. The name of the place is Seven Wonders. People who live there have mental problems. They have spent years in psychiatric hospital and are registered with a psychiatrist and community psychiatric nurse. In May 1996, I stayed there for one-week assessment. I did not let a new venture frighten me as it will open up many new doors for me, and will certainly bring more contentment to my life. It will soon be my time to do well. A little patience and it will all work out for the best. It was quite pleasant and I was able to relax without anybody troubling me. Peace and harmony was mine for the taking. I had good reason to celebrate leaving home. I achieved what I wanted. I did it by hurting myself. I took an overdose something drastic that happened got me out of the house I grew up in because it was an ambition of mine to get out of there.
My vision was not an illusion. Spending time in hospital was not a waste of time.

DARKENED LIGHT

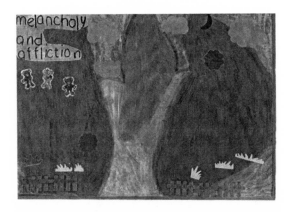

I came to a crossroads and headed for the hills. Moving to Blackburn is a new environment and change in my domestic situation. I wanted to break free from my family. I needed to procreate the difference how I live and how I would like to live. It will improve my psychological health. Subconsciously I wanted comfort and tenderness. I wanted to let loose and have some fun. Find a willingness to view the world from a different point.

Mental Health Teams ate the referral point through sources gain access to the specialist service to move into residential care. Specialist services should review my needs at least every six months. A care plan would be prepared, social support provided by the rehabilitation team. A single plan, which sets contributions and a single key worker, will keep in touch with me, and make sure that all the elements of care is carried out. The approach is jointly between the Mental Health Team and rehabilitation should dovetail with care management in Social Services.

Care programs need to be up to date and have review dates. A psychiatrist has not assessed me but Hilda and Benjamin will keep on doing so at intervals to see whether my care programs is going to plan because of people in authority deciding what is best. What kind of support I needed did not take Hilda and Benjamin long to decide. Hilda and Benjamin are one of the most important groups of professionals providing mental health care for me. A key worker will undertake much of the direct work.

In meetings with care, workers Hilda and Benjamin should give feedbacks on how far I have gone with my targets. Strategic agreement between social services and mental health teams are necessary to qualify me for a grant essential to move into Local Authority Housing They provided care because of funds between health and services. Hilda and Benjamin think I need to be in care settings I have less series mental health problems. They took notice of me because steps are required to improve my life. Hilda and Benjamin need my participation in key decisions.

SUSAN SPLAINE

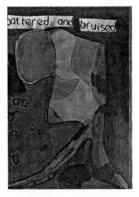

The road I am on now will lead to what is looming over the horizon. After careful consideration, I will decide what my opportunities are. I made the decisions I made because of bad luck. Embark upon new and successful plans. I want to gain satisfaction from all of my activities.

<u>RULES</u> <u>AND</u> <u>RESPONSIBILITIES</u>

1) On admission residents will talk through a therapeutic programmed designed to meet their individual needs are expected to take part in all activities specified on their programmed.

2) Residents are expected to engage willingly in the process of rehabilitation and be available to work on their programmed from 9am - 5pm Monday to Friday, there *may* also be activities arranged during the evenings and at weekends.

3) Residents are required to be up and dressed by 9am in order to begin work on their programmed. At weekends, it a house rules **to** be awake before 11.30am.

4) All residents must attend the morning meeting in the group room at
9.15 am on weekdays after collecting their medication from the main office

5) No television before 12.30pm.Noise kept to a reasonable level at all times.

6) When a new resident arrives or when visitors come residents should be polite and friendly.

7) Any form of violence or threat of violence to others or damage to property is forbidden as is the use of insulting or disrespectful language or behaviour.

8) If you self-harm or become self-destructive, we will put you into hospital.

9) We do not want residents to bring sharp objects into the house such as knifes and blades. Kitchen knives are available from staff on request.

10) The consumption of alcohol on the premises or during any organised activity s not allowed. It is a house rule not to go out drinking or come back intoxicated.

Residents who have alcohol problems will receive counseling.

11) It is a house rule not to use any unauthorized medication, illegal drugs or chemicals.

12) It is a house rule not to bring any sexually explicit or pornographic material onto the premises.

13) It is a house rule not to engage in any romantic and/ or sexual relationships with other residents.

14) Each resident is responsible for ensuring that there is no buying or selling of goods with other residents or staff members.
It is a house rule not to lend or borrow money.

15) It is a house rule not to buy gifts for members of staff.

16) It is a house rule to engage in any illegal or antisocial behavior, which may have a detrimental effect on themselves, other residents and staff, or members of the public.

17) Residents may only use such personal belongings as computers, CB radio and musical instruments after prior consultation with the manager.

18) Residents not allowed pets on the premises.

19) Residents must read fire instructions carefully and follow all fire safety procedures promptly when the fire alarm sounds. It is a house rule not to smoking in bedrooms and the use of candles in any area of the building.

20) It is a house rule to support each other by confronting irresponsible, unhealthy or harmful behavior, which they may observe, and report any breach rules by any residents to a member of staff.

21) Residents who are leaving must be responsible for taking all their personal belongings with them.

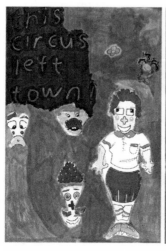 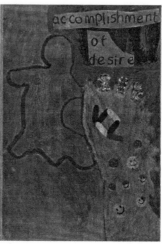

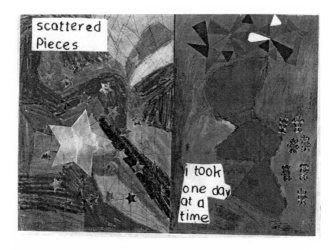

CHAPTER SIX

On June 10 1996 was the day I had a new lease of life and able to build my life back up on my misfortunes. I felt smug, overjoyed, felt like doing heal kicks. Hilda and Benjamin picked me up in the morning loaded the car with my bags, nobody said goodbye. Driving to Blackburn, I reflected on the events that got me out of that house and into residential care. The main factor why I needed help was because I needed help to develop social skills and communicate with people, what got me out is I took an overdose because of a sex attack. That made social workers stands up and takes notice of a person in despair.

From the outside of the building, it looks like a big house. Inside there are four flats with a single bedroom, a double bedroom kitchen and lounge. There are also two single flats. Downstairs on the bottom floor is the office, kitchen dining and group room is in one room where we had morning **meetings**, people who do not make their own meals in the flats can have a member of staff help them cook in the kitchen. The laundry room is downstairs, so is the office, a bedroom where night staff sleep and three storage cupboards.

Ezekiel and Rojo are married they own Seven Wonders. Stella does administration work in the office. Oscar and Hope two other staff members are involved in a relationship. They are therapists. There were four key workers, Jancis, Angus, Joe and Misty, another support worker Brent *and Scott* who later on left for a job working with computers. Dorinda was a student social worker. Claribel helps residents find a flat when they are ready to move on. She also visited them as a community support worker.

Seven Wonders also run three other homes. The next step for some residents is to move into a terraced house near the infirmary hospital on Webster Street. Four people can live there it is more independent living. Jeremiah and Tukishi work there but they do not sleep over. There are also two old people's homes; one of them is Final Resting Place. I do not know the name of the other one but it is near the local shops near Seven

Wonders.

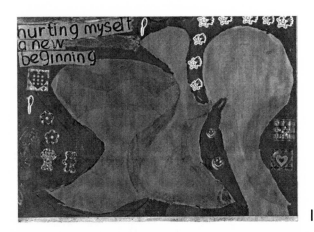

I shared a flat with Nadia who lived there for over a year Wanda moved in a couple weeks after me on the same day Nadia went on holiday to Morecambe Bay with other residents Jancis and Claribel. My mum found out where I lived because Benjamin gave her a Seven Wonders leaflet, at the back of it is a map how to get there from the train station. (Seven Wonders is in walking distance of the Train Station). I felt surprised because I expected not to see her again. Oscar took her into the office said I might not want to see her.

Abbey put my ten thousand pounds compensation into the bank in Sale when it came in the post at the house because I did not give my change of address. I thought a lot about the acquisition. I had catalogue debts to pay off, book and music club debts. Ezekiel advised me to put eight thousand pounds into an interest account. On my **own,** I would not have taken care because I saw it has 'blood money' and wanted to burn it. The money tided me over because I got £15 shopping money and £14 spending money.

When I went out on shopping sprees Ezekiel got stressed and fretful because he is money minded. I saw old clothes as rubbish so threw them out. In a review meeting with Hilda and Benjamin my finances was the only thing they were concerned about, I did not stand my ground by telling them my personal well-being should be of most importance. Most of the residents had different benefits to me, so they got more than £14 a week.

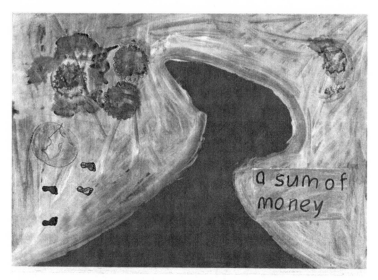

On Monday morning, *I* went food shopping.

DARKENED LIGHT

Afterwards I went for just the one drink in the pub. On Tuesday afternoon, I went out for a drive with one of the groups. We either went to a cafe in town for a coffee, sometimes we went to a pub for a coffee. On Wednesday at the local college a part of the mental health One Step Course, a qualified instructor took two residents, me, and Joe the support worker came with us and other people on outdoor pursuit's course. On Thursday afternoon, I went to relaxation classes with Misty and other residents. On Friday afternoon, residents at Webster Street and Seven Wonders went out with about four staff members in their cars.

Pleasant company cheered me up. It seemed contagious that everybody had a good time. I did not want to antagonize anyone but there was a coming together between me and other people. I became good friends with Sandy I am seven months older than she is. Joe the support worker was the first person I built up a relationship with, drawn to him because of retort and his good sense of humour. Wanda had a good relationship with Nadia that made me feel cut off because I did not have a sense of belonging. I could not initiate conversation with any of them. I would not respond to Wanda when she was being nosy because I am secretive. Asking what I am eating reminded of all the year's when Jasmine said every day" what are you eating". Wanda would lose her temper because I did not explain to her why I hate people asking me what I am eating. I went out to the pub to give her some breathing space to calm down because she got so irate.

Nadia was like a daughter to Rojo, they had a close relationship. When Rojo was not around Nadia missed her. She showed it by having a glum expression, feeling down and fretted because she wanted her and only her to talk-to-talk. There was a lot of physical affection between them. They gave each other cuddles and sat close together on the sofa. Rojo sometimes had meals in the flat with her. Nadia was the special one who everyone loved and adored. I found it a strain living with Wanda and Nadia. I did not click with either of them. I was not content to potter around the flat with them. I got headaches, my nose and throat felt congested because they smoked a lot.

In the evening downstairs in the kitchen residents played dominos if they wanted to, it was compulsory for me mixing with people. Every morning we had to get up at 9.00 am to go to the morning meetings. It was about appointments, people had during the day and activities going on. We got our mail from the office residents also had their morning medication in the office. If somebody did not get out of bed for the meetings the staff, would either ring their flat on the internal phone or go to their rooms, to get them out of bed. Nadia did not have to go to the meetings if she did not want to. Jancis and Claribel made her a cup of coffee and took it to her in her bedroom.

DARKENED LIGHT

It took a few weeks for Angus to do a programmed with me as a result I got very bored, because I would not leave the house on my own. I drank because I was bored. I brought cans of Wood Pecker Cider from the off license, drank walking the street. Oscar has worked in clinics working with alcoholics. Hilda and Benjamin told him I have a drink problem. It was part of my treatment at some point I should have counseling with Oscar.

People cannot seem to cope with abuse they suffered as children and by husbands; it is memories that make people unwell. Most of them live in the past and feel sorry for them. I cope because I am a cold on the inside sort of person. People suffered from mental illness and psychological problems. We all must accept that our life needs to change and never carry on being the same. Life has not been going right for any of us that are why we are in psychiatric care. I thought support workers could read my mind when I needed help so very quietly just sat there. We had to go to them whenever we were upset. I made the effort to reach out because others were aware of my needs.

I took the chance, a fresh set of circumstances to take a turn for the better. I was wise and had faith. Each day was a bridge between the past and the future. Nothing stays the same forever. I looked forward with hope and optimism on this road I hoped I would get to where I wanted to go eventually. I expected big changes. I wanted to make life much brighter. I needed to liven up my personality. I will come to realize that changes will bring out the best in me.

Angus was my key worker. From the outset, I could not form a relationship with Angus that was easy going and stress free. He behaved like a dominion because he was in a position of authority. He was not somebody I felt comfortable with talking to about deep-seated feelings when I wanted to be serious. During our sessions, if I felt frustrated I went to the pub afterwards. What we discussed and talked about was always about him, what he wants from me, what he wants me to do. I did find myself disagreeing with him. I felt like something inside was going to explode. Living at Seven Wonders day to day is set out to be structured Angus talked about with me what I should do every day but he had the last say and what is best for me. I did not need him to go shopping with me. I did not want to do a shopping list. I did not like swimming. Angus put pressure on me to engage in conversations by asking questions.

I was sometimes reluctant to spend too much time socializing. When it was just a one-way conversation, the staff got very disappointed. I felt bad about myself because of their stern attitude. I did not make the effort socially when I felt low I just wanted to be left alone when I showed social isolation. I did not maintain a sense of balance with my moods. When I was emotionally high giddiness, outburst of laughter and elation would come over me. I found it all very frustrating with every step forward I took three steps back.

I was there to develop social skills it seemed like staff members wanted me to talk non-stop. Angus gave me a telling off when I felt tired, unhappy and bored. He told me if I do not do my programmed then find somewhere else to live. I did not focus on the here and now! The only way I will be able to enrich my life, is eliminate what has been robbing me of my peace of mind. I focus far too much on minor details and neglect the wider picture.

Hope took me to the doctors so I could register with *Dr Kern my* new GP. At nine and half stone, I was the right weight for my height. Counseling with Hope was about my childhood, what caused my anxiety. I have a communication problem because of my fear of speaking. I was worried people laughed at me when they heard me speak. I used one word rather than an entire sentence. I avoided conversations because my mouth trembled. I was nervous so it made me stutter. *Anxiety* affected my behavior and impaired performance.

Upsets also made my life difficult! I tried talking about my bad times and traumas. Hope told me that I feel sorry for myself and to forget about it but it was ok for everybody else to be upset because of bad memories. I have not had the chance to talk about that feeling of emptiness because I feel cheated of time. I wanted to use time for reflection. On August 30 1994, a change took place in me. *Images* are difficult to dismiss from my mind. There is a dark side to me that was the driving force putting self in a vulnerable position I do not feel guilty because it was a cold and selfish thing to do.

I did not find Hope or Angus a source of support. They told me that I do not suffer from depressive moods. I felt as if I could not carry on or face another day. I had suicidal thoughts. The only thought that kept me going I want some good times before I die. Memories from the past did weigh heavily on my mind. I felt physically ill because I was not confiding in anyone, as there was not anyone to talk to, because my thinking process did not matter. I had counseling to help me form relationships with people I felt comfortable with because there were residents who I could not relate too. I wanted to progress, grow and flourish naturally. I found it an uphill struggle to regain composure and tranquility. I failed to realize that on occasions the best time is the present. I needed to get into the habit of looking for the positive aspect, when I find it I need to continue to look at it rather than looking at the leaden grey parts. It will help me through the rough patches.

When I felt lazy because I was going through a

period of despondency all I wanted was to be alone. I spent time on my own in my bedroom. I wrote down my thoughts, feelings and sentiments. I had a vision in my mind seeing life as a journey on my earthly adventures. I used sentiments to describe the earth in a symbolic way of expression. I felt out of sorts so I mindlessly cast aside troubles. I tended to be secretive, mysterious, reserved and introverted. I am not always honest with myself or other people. I shut them out because I was unsure of how I felt. Life seemed grey and unexciting. When my mum came to see me for the second time, I went clothes shopping. Wanda who is a thief stole £20 from my purse I kept in my bedroom draw. I told Ezekiel about it all he said is I cannot prove it was she, but he had a talk to her

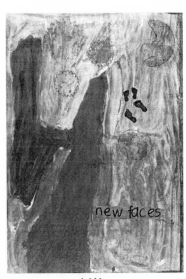

new faces

I moved into flat four with Noreen who was in her mid thirties. Julie had just moved out who she shared a bedroom with, into Final Resting Place, even though she was not much older than Toby who also lived there. He was in the psychiatric ward. I slept in his single room until he came out off the psychiatric hospital. I shared with Noreen in the double room. I adapted quickly to my new flat. I put extra effort into my appearance. I went to the hairdressers and changed my hairstyle.

I felt much more comfortable within myself and sought out the companies of fresh faces. I feel resentment towards Mother Nature because if I did not have my mum's genetics I would not have seen myself as a freak. I lived in a dream world that I have a Mexican mother, and American father and come from an upper class family. I did precious little to be centre of attention. I stayed adaptable so I would have been ready to move forward with the times. When life changes good luck might come my way when I have ambitions and goals I want to chase.

In my own time, I hoped I would resolve inner fears and frustrations. Find greater emotional stability and happiness. I hoped I would be less inclined to suffer in silence. I wanted to feel more stable, at peace within myself. I have the will power to readjust my focus. Engage in activities instead of feeling like banging my head against a brick wall, and pulling my hair out. I want to reclaim my life, build it back up the way I want it to be. I want to feel joy, laugh, close to people and feel confident.

Noreen is absent-minded: she was untidy in the kitchen it was always a mess and dirty. I am self-conscious about hygiene in the kitchen. Toby was in harmony as Noreen. They did not take pride if the flat was dirty or clean. They did not have high standards. I felt anger towards them and carried resentment around inside me. I got very moody and felt miserable. I had a preference to be alone because I found it hard to believe anybody cared because I lived in a pigsty. I became disinclined to make an effort with housework. I felt very low because of them and believed things would not improve. I lost my appetite. I lost weight. I could not sleep. I stopped making meals for myself in a dirty kitchen. I lived on crackers, biscuits, salad and bread. I accepted that how I felt was quite reasonable under the circumstances.

I did not have a bath regularly.
I did not clean, cut toe, or fingernails.
I did not brush my hair.
I slept during the day.
I did not express emotions.
I did my own laundry but I did separate white clothes from colour clothes.
I put my clothes in the wardrobe.
I did not iron.
I washed my own dishes.

I mop the kitchen floor.
I did not make my bed.
I like bathrooms to be clean.
I am well organized.

The relationship between Rojo and I was not a good one! We did not even talk. She always gave me a sly look when I passed her by up and down the corridor, up and down the stairs. She gave me stone cold looks. She smiled at me maliciously. I found it hurtful as if she was intimidating me. She was the last person I would go to when on the verge of desperation. I wanted to leave, but it was not up to me to decide when I want to move out. I had to endure her attitude towards me, bide my time until I move on. I did not see myself strong enough to leave just yet! I did not know where my life was heading. I could not see it staying the way it was.

I think it was bad luck for me, Hilda and Benjamin chose Seven Wonders. It was an unpleasant surprise how Rojo was with me. My world was imperfect there! I was too frightened to approach her. I looked up to the black rain cloud over in a place where I wanted it to stop raining because I thought I found my paradise: instead hell on earth. Compounded by her attitude I hoped to gain good fortune out of this adversity. I was isolated and alone to deal with her because Hilda and Benjamin thought Seven Wonders is a good place. Other staff members were not aware what was going on.

I needed somebody on my side to talk to about her. I knew what to expect from Social Workers. They would have sat us all down in a small dark room and talk about it. They think talking can solve everything when my life situation needed to change non-verbal abusing me. Reporting her, making a complaint, I still would have found myself trapped there. It would not have changed a thing but make the situation more intense. I dismissed her completely. It was the best thing I could have done to rise above it, detach myself from her. It was a long-standing difficulty to get on with the rest of my life.

I was not doing activities I enjoyed doing. I felt like hardly anything was worthwhile. There simply was no urgency to get something started or completed. I ended up doing little or nothing. I wanted to avoid doing some of the activities because of lack of enthusiasm. Seeing life as dull made me feel isolated.

Feeling the need to reach the toilet quickly caused me distress. Psychological problems and stress disturbed my bladder control. It had a physical and emotional affect on me. Feeling of uneasiness anxious, tense, worried and nervous made me go to the toilet every thirty minutes during the daytime. At night, whilst I was trying to sleep I went to the toilet about seven times. My family doctor arranged before I moved to Seven

Wonders, to see a Specialist at Withington Hospital. I had a cystoscopy: It is an observation of inside of the bladder using a telescope. There was not anything physically wrong with me. It is something that would phase out when my anxiety level is not as high.

I began to hate going out on the Friday afternoon activities because I found activities we did boring. I got tension headaches on Fridays because Misty and Angus put pressure on me by saying it is the taking part that counts. It was always about them what they want to do. Misty was the one who arranged Friday afternoon trips out. Gave me a hard time when I was not in a good mood. When I felt happy, I do not know why I was happy, because I did not have anything to be happy about because I saw life as being dull, even though I had grand plans. I think Angus and Misty found it confusing why one minute I was in a good mood; wake up in the morning after about two weeks of happiness and my mood is black. When I was in a dark horrible place feeling so far apart from everybody, I did not talk about it in order to avoid adding confusion that surrounded my situation. I should of aired my views and get my feelings of resentment and hatred out. I do not have any manners but I do try to be polite just to keep the peace. I felt ashamed when a big group of us went into a café and took up all of the seats.

DARKENED LIGHT

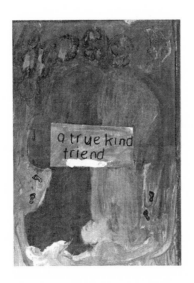

In December 1996, I started to have counseling sessions with Oscar about my drinking. Ezekiel saw me drinking in the street, when he drove down the road. I had not been talking to anybody, about what is it I want how I really do feel. I could describe what was happening inside my mind a secret I was keeping to myself. Muddled thoughts gave me mental tension and made the day drag. I found it a waste of time talking about my physical ill health, because they told me it is just anxiety. They are wrong so wrong if only they knew.

I did not want to make changes or give, up the bottle because I resented everybody telling me what is best for me. Deep down I think there is much more to my mental health than just anxiety and social skills. Sometimes I feel like I am somebody else. I think my inner self was beginning to come out the side to me that have been repressive since childhood. I do not get drunk, so it did not give *me* heartache because I did not feel guilty. It is the pleasure and enjoyment I get from it every time I felt like a drink. Going to the pub got me out of the house. Since June, I have not approached my problem situation about longing for a much better life.

I want to prosper and fly away like a butterfly. I want to live in a nice house and go on holidays. I will not trap myself in relationships with people I do not get on with, love or like. It does not have to be a boyfriend. I trap myself inside a fantasyland so I have not approached my feelings of deadness and emptiness in a different way so that the outcome if change will ever take place will have a positive effect on my every day life. I drink because of a brief encounter I had with Alex. He could have been my soul mate if we got it together. Rejection as a child did not make me drink. I did not drink because of desperation, what I did to get out of that house. I did not drink large amounts before Roxy was not in my life anymore. I drank more because I trapped myself inside a fantasyland about Alex and me. I told Oscar I have not been *drinking* when *I.* had. I did not stick to giving up when it was not so easy. I did not give it more time.

I do not think I am not capable of recovery from dependence on alcohol. I did not make the decision of actually wanting to give up. I found letting go hard work it is not an easy thing to do. Letting out my secret will be my first step on new ground old memories do not taint. Then I might make a commitment to myself, stick to it no matter how hard it turns out to be. It would be a chance to recover from not to be dependent on alcohol.

RELAPSE PREVENTION

Taking responsibility for Rehabilitation or recovering also means taking responsibility for ensuring that Relapse does not occur. Relapse to fall back. I felt as if I have missed something. Relapse is an event and a process. Relapse is not an accident it is a block in awareness. Something I could not admit to or blanked out, for relapse to occur. The effect of relapse is loss of self-worth, guilt, remorse, disheartened at having failed again, a conviction that things will never improve.

THE PROCESS OF RELAPSE

Ego –Complacency – The mask I am fine. Denial one slip will not matter. I had secret thoughts about not giving up so I relapsed.

I avoided facing my dark secret.
I did not justify my drinking by rationalization.

127

I was dishonest because of distortion of the truth, also dishonest by omission.

I did not share anger or resentment.

Wanting too much too soon is being impatient.

Frustration: Things may not go my way.

Fear Apprehension about well-being.

Depression: I hate being alone but I do have tendencies towards loneliness, isolating and defensive.

Idle day dreaming and lost of constructive living will make you not want to give up.

Irregular eating/sleeping can make a person relapse.

Development of "I do not care" attitude because you still want to drink.

Unrealistic expectations of myself did not make me drink.

Re-entry to the world can make a drunk feel lost and lonely, and vulnerable. Behaving in a different way that made you, drink may not have immediate effect so a drunk can become disenchanted and disheartened, and return quickly to the bottle. Every time I left the house, I compared myself with young women who had children. I also compared myself with children who looked miserable; I thought to myself I'm glad that isn't me. I do not pity myself because I live in hope my fortunes will change. Open rejection of help. The denial, distortion, rationalizing, delusions can cause a change in a drunks emotional response. Problems and conflicts might arise with family and friends. How a person is behaving externally can come across as being dysfunctional.

Life problems are continually re-created. Relapse prevention is intervening earlier in the process. Start talking and sharing honestly before things build up into a crisis.

Talking about my anger, despair and anxiety I needed to open up, and consider the problems that brought me to treatment. The relationship between Oscar and I is a way of experiencing, and recognizing the appropriate ways I relate to people. The insight gained allowed me to develop more appropriate ways of relating now, rather than staying in the protective but limiting ways I learnt in childhood. The aim of therapy is to increase self-esteem by making me feel valued, accepted even when I reveal the parts of myself I hate. I do not like speaking because of bad genetics it affects the way that I think and how I behave, because I keep myself isolated. Thoughts such as I never get anything right. Nobody will ever love me. It affects both my mood and how I behave.

Hilda and Benjamin had a review meeting with the senior staff at Seven Wonders and Angus. I did not want to sit in it because it would have sent shivers up and down my spine. I do not like praise. I did not want to listen to everybody talking about my progress. They were pleased that I attended worthless Step One Courses at the local College. I did sports and music when I cannot even play instruments or write songs.   The lessons seemed like they were never ending because I was not interested or enthused.

My mum brought me a lot of chocolate for Christmas. She also brought me Christmas shopping and toiletries. Some of the residents at Seven Wonders spent Christmas with their families. I spent Christmas at Seven Wonders. On Christmas Eve, we had a party there. Brent organized it and Joe slept over. I think it was at the party I spoke to Brent for the first time. I sometimes brushed passed him in a bad mood and he would say how I am feeling. Christmas Day Hope and Oscar cooked the meal. I had nut roast and vegetables. I got a mobile charm for my Christmas present. On Boxing Day, we went to watch an ice skating show at the local theatre. New Years Eve we had a party at Seven Wonders. Residents from final resting place came to the party.

SUKEY LILY
SEVEN WONDERS REVIEW
19 DECEMBER 1996

Sukey has continued to make good progress with rehabilitation programmed.
Sukey has an adaptable nature so it did not take long for her to be at ease with both staff and residents and began to initiate contact spontaneously.
Sukey continues to be involved in house activities. She attends the morning meetings, swimming

group, Relaxation Group, and the Friday afternoon activity group.

She has regularly attended the Step one stone courses at the local college in computers, music and sports and plans to continue this programmed in the New Year.

Finances

Sukey followed advice from the Finance Manager at Seven Wonders and the Manager at her bank. She has invested a large part of her capital.

Closed downs key's accounts with catalogues because she has paid of her debts.

MEDICATION

Sukey is not currently taking any prescribed medication.

General health

Sukey has had a number of courses of antibiotics over the past three months prescribed by her doctor for E.N.T. infections. She attended Withington Hospital on 11 October 1996 for an investigation under anesthetic after she repeatedly complained to her doctor about gynecological problems. She has a further appointment for the results of this investigation on 21 January 1997

Further Development

Sukey has made good progress forming relationships with members of staff. She remains highly motivated to her rehabilitation. She continues to need high levels of support and this expected to continue for the near future.

Sukey has been addressing personal issues in her

counseling sessions for some time, but has also recently asked for a programmed which will assist her in dealing with her problems relating to alcohol dependency.

Good self-esteem means good self-confidence. You have a positive self-picture, with a strong awareness of your personal needs. You have a real sense of your own significance and value. You are able to cope with and learn from negative experiences. Improved self-confidence: If you feel confident, both your verbal and body language match up and convince people of your sincerity. You will not tolerate put downs or unfairness. You challenge people calmly but firmly.

Self-confidence: You are able to be assertive about your needs, to ask questions, to make choices, decisions and to be tenacious. You have enough confidence to listen well to others and respond to their rights and needs. Better self-esteem: People treat you with respect, listen to you and seek out your opinion, you feel even more valued, which enhances your self-image further.

Poor self-esteem means: You have a negative self-picture with little awareness of needs. Low self-worth leads to feelings of insignificance. Negative setbacks or comments tend to overly disappoint or

distress you.
Outer Self-Confidence: Poor relationship skills: You feel passive and flustered because of a growing mismatch between what you say and body language, which reads as fear and anxiety.

Low self-confidence: Unable to clear or direct about expressing my needs and wants. Fear of failure and lack of confidence means you fail to challenge authority or ask questions, are easily deterred when things go wrong.
Lower self-esteem: You see other people as not considering your feelings because you are a sensitive weak person who cries easily when upset. Your self-image is further weakened and self-evaluation as a person of respect.

I NEED TO DEVELOP ASSERTIVENESS CHARACTERISTICS

Communicating your needs clearly is an assertive interpersonal skill. It describes a way of communicating my needs, my wants, my feelings to people without infringing their rights. It means acknowledging my own rights, whilst respecting the rights of other people. The nature of my problem is seeing me as a freak. I did not discuss seeing myself as a freak in counseling sessions. Therefore, I have not overcome my problem not liking communicating with people. I just want to be silent forever. I sometimes wish I were born deaf. When it comes to communicating, I do not think I will not ever build up my self-confidence. Writing my book, hoping to get it published is my only goal in life. I think it is realistic because I do not see why it will not happen. Books about Mental Health do appeal to people.

I will not ever be more effective with people: I feel good about myself because I have artistic intelligence and a good imagination. I do not let people take advantage of me because I take advantage of situations to better myself or because I like danger and trouble. I come across as having innocence about me, but I do not. I did not keep myself out of dangerous situations because I went out looking for something risky to happen to me. When a man picks me up in the street I like playing games with him, by giving the wrong impressions, because all I want from him is to buy the drinks. I say no without feeling guilty because I do not have a conscience. I do not have serenity. I change my mind because I can think for myself. I make mistakes and do not blame anybody else for my failings. I live and learn from mistakes and accidents. I say I do not know. I do not understand. I do not care. I ask people for what I need help and support with, whilst realizing that person has the right to say no. I am a cold person. I am not very sympathetic so I choose weather or not to get involved in the problems of somebody else. I please myself before I please others.

DARKENED LIGHT

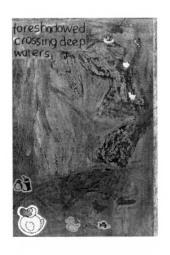

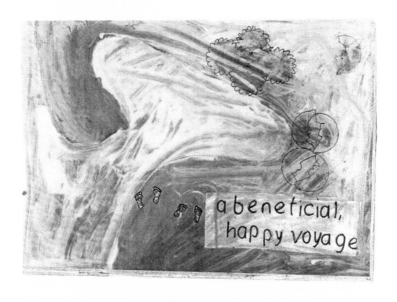

SUSAN SPLAINE

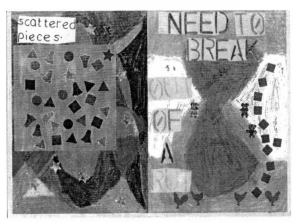

CHAPTER SEVEN

In January ninety-ninety-seven, I put a keep fit plan together with Angus. We went jogging, joined a gym. Exercise played an essential part in maintaining strength, endurance. Exercise is important for physical health. It is also a very good way of relaxing and relieving stress. It increases the release of endorphins, a brain chemical that releases the feeling of euphoria.

For along period I am without feeling joy or excitement. I feel just sadness, hurting inside and pain. Deep sadness does last a long time. Hidden anger and resentment caused me a great deal of damage. It made me feel withdrawn and unhappy, feeling like that. I get many physical symptoms I feel like I cannot cope with it.

During the day time when I felt down my mood lifted at night. I eat more during the evening. I have more energy because of it I get restless. I go out walking because I cannot keep still. I get tingling sensations in my legs and back. I get sore throats at least every five weeks. I get tension headaches. I have sleepless nights. I have many thoughts going round inside my head. Neck and scalp muscles cause headaches above my eyes. I get tension in my neck and scalp. I felt achy over the top of my skull and neck. My head felt heavy and scalp muscles sore. When I did not have an appetite, I felt nauseated in the morning. I got a sickening heaviness in the pit of my stomach. When I felt weak, I thought my legs were going to snap. I got tension in my leg muscles and a sore back. My legs felt shaky. I got blurred vision. I felt giddy and breathless. I went to the toilet frequently.

Over the weekend, I felt a lot of anxiety facing a confrontation with Ezekiel and Hope because of my foolish behaviour. I felt like I let them down and disappointed them because I do not learn from mistakes; if only they knew I have been drinking with **men** I had just met fireworks will go off. On Sunday, I was meant to go out to church with Mormons but not allowed out. I wanted to lash out but I did not. I felt like I was locked inside a prison cell. I want to he more liberal and freer to make my own decisions. On Monday, Hope and Ezekiel confronted me because I got myself involved in an unhealthy situation. The two Mormons I met up with Shane looked just like Milton. Inside my mind, I drifted back to ninety-ninety-four. On that same evening, I went out with Steve and Shane to visit an elderly man at his flat, who I had already met fortunately for me he was not in so I went back to Seven Wonders. I did not feel at ease with going into somebody's flat, even though I chose to go with two men. Ezekiel was working late in the office I told him that I did not go into the flat. I will stop seeing the Mormons. He was pleased that I came to my senses and gave him peace of mind because he worried about me.

I like nature and wildlife, horticulture so on September 25 ninety-ninety- seven I decided to do a Biology Course at Blackburn College. It was at six pm every Thursday until nine 0'clock pm. I stopped going because at some point I want to study horticulture full time, not just one night a week. Horticulture was my ambition when I was about fifteen. I could not go to college because of discouragement from Jasmine, Paddy, and my mum who put me down and dented my confidence

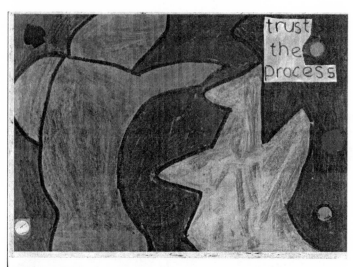

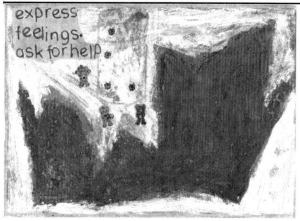

THE REHABILIATION PROCESS

Rehabilitation is not a single event it is a series of different events, over a period of time, which add up to a complete process.

TRUST THE PROCESS
If a person does not believe and trust in their programmed, then it will not **work for** them. Strengthen their trust and belief in the programmed at Seven Wonders.

Rehabilitation means making changes. These changes include:

Confused -Confident
Insecure - Secure
Unstable -Stable
Isolated - Social
Aggressive-Assertive
Self-harming-Self-respect
Pain- Pleasure

Aims: To resolve **problems** Too **plan, and build, a better future**
What is your plan is your plan?
Nothing changes if nothing changes.

NEEDS

 Value, meaning and purpose make you worthy as a person self-worth.
 To achieve what I want is power.

Thought, action and choice give you freedom.
Pleasure, variety and creativity you get enjoyment
from having fun.

My attitude is to relate to my self and other
people. Respect for myself and   other people.
My behaviour is to be healthy and grow. If I were
irresponsible, it would make me unhealthy and
self-defeating. Choices and consequences of my
behaviour and attitude is my responsibility
because of my attitude.

Since living in Blackburn, I had met some vulgar
men. On a Sunday **afternoon,** I met an Asian Man
in the Town Centre. I sat on a bench drinking a
strawberry milkshake. He **initiated** conversation
offered to take me to the cinema so I hung around
with him. We went *for a* walk and walked past a
taxi office he held my hand because he wanted to
show me of to a mate who worked there. We went
to get something to eat, fries. He brought me two
lots of fries because he thought I was thin. We
went into the Town Centre car park where he
pulled his pants down and started masturbating. I
ran away, went home. We ended up not going to
the cinema, he did not promise so I was not
disappointed.

I did not *give* anybody my address or the phone
number of the office at Seven Wonders. If a man
phoned me up the *staff* would have interrogated
my unhealthy behaviour. I did not want **to make a**
long—standing change about how I made myself

vulnerable with men, I saw it as a pleasure moment.

I kept shilly-shally a secret because I did not have the strength or resources to face a showdown with Ezekiel, Rojo, Oscar and Hope. I came across to them as being such a good girl who **is not any trouble. Deep down inside I do not see somebody who is so sweet and innocent.**

I did not want to get involved in a relationship with somebody I did not feel affection for because it will make me feel miserable. I want to see passion burning in a man's eyes. The men I came across I was not physically attracted to them. Life is not much fun on your own. All I want is somebody to take me out in the evenings. My mind was preoccupation with alcohol. I made the decision I did not want to stop drinking. I did not take steps to change because I did not express regrets about my drinking. I met Asian lads who do not drink but brought me drinks. I went swimming on my own because I thought it might make me feel much more comfortable wearing a swimming costume. An Asian lad spoke to me in the pool. When I got out, he told me to wait for him, so I did. I let him walk me home but he lost interest because of where I lived.

I did not see eye to eye with Angus about how I felt life being slow moving. All that mattered to him is that I am doing worthless step one classes. I needed to break out of a rut. I needed something to believe in and hold on to as well as my fortune journey in life. I needed something to be passionate about that is the driving force that gives you motivation to work towards goals. Nothing was not there for me to achieve besides finishing my book. I got very frustrated because I had the desire to achieve something, but nothing to aim for. It could take years before I finish my book.

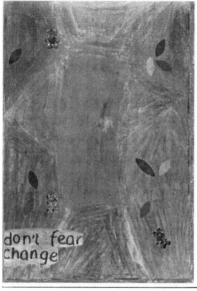
don't fear change

Angus and Hope told me that I am not ready to make concrete plans, so I did not talk my differences through with them. I told me I am not ready to do something constructive. I have to be much more sociable first: Visit people in their flats. Talk more and play games, scrabble and dominos. I did not overcome my unpleasantness feeling fed up all day. I moved into flat five because the double room converted into two single rooms. Carman spent most of her time in her bedroom. She had meals cooked for her downstairs in the kitchen. I had the kitchen in the flat to myself so I had the time to make gourmet meals for my self I had nobody rushing me because they wanted to make their meals. The only programmed Carman watched on television was top of the pops. She shouted aloud at the staff when she felt annoyed and frustrated. Once she went out with the Friday group and cried all afternoon. I was the one who had to comfort her. She would not leave my side. I had a headache because I found it stressful going out in such a big group. It was hard to decide whom to talk to or spend time with because there were too many people. Carman did not go on the camping holidays. Her favorite pastime was going out to Marks & Spencer everyday. On Thursday night, she went out to the YMCA disco with Noreen and Kane. I sometimes went with them. Rodney also lived in flat five; he spent most of his time in flat two with Wanda because she was the love of his life. I got on with Carman. She liked to give me cuddles. Every day said how lovely I am. Rodney still went out shopping brought tinned food never eaten by him. He only drank milk and coffee when Wanda came round to the flat for a drink I do not think he never drank a full carton of milk.

I had my own kitchen cutely and utensils in boxes and plastic draws because there was not enough room in the kitchen cupboards. There was one cupboard for food. There was one cupboard in the kitchen for cutely. One cupboard for detergents, cleaning sponges, clothes. My mum brought me the video she did not want because she brought a new one.

How I feel stir up emotions I thought were long gone. Being naive, childlike I want to feel loved, security and a stranger to become my friend. I am blunt because I am too trusting. Feelings of inferiority and inadequacy eradicated until certain changes begin from within me. Despite my behavioral problems, I do have some good qualities I am not putting too use:

I do have good common sense.
I dream up ideas.
I am interested in things that interest me.
I enjoy nature; seeing things grow and prosper.
I want to live a harmonious and successful life.

In July ninety-ninety-seven my mum, sisters Abbey and Jasmine, her new boyfriend Sidney came to see me. Jasmine met Sidney at Rochdale Market where they both worked on two different vegetables stalls. Her ex- fiancé was still Jasmine's boss. They lived in a bed-sit over a pub called the Bulls Head. Ironically, we went to the Moorings pub near the canal where I mostly hung out. I had vegetable burger and chips to eat for my meal. I did not drink any alcohol I told them that I am having counseling. I had already decided to bend the rules before I signed the contract. On that same day, residents had communal meals together at the weekend. I went back there had something to eat because vegetarian food brought for me.

I did not get the help I needed to break out of the cycle I was in I did feel physically unwell a lot especially with headaches, sore throats and stiff legs. I got into a mixed state of emotions. What I want is peace and contentment. I needed to talk about what goes on inside me, admit my feelings to my self. Share them with somebody who will listen to me. Feelings come from my needs not measured up to. I get feelings like those that I cannot go through all that again. I really cannot but I do go through it. When I am very tired, I cannot face a big meal. I eat nuts, dried fruit and fresh fruit. It is difficult in setback to remember how well I felt. When I make good- progress I rush through jobs that needs doing. When with a big group I can enjoy myself. When my energy is high, I keep myself active because it makes the day go by quickly. I go through a phase when the days are somewhat sluggish because of the stop and go feel to it. I had early nights when I could not wait for the day to end.

I was reluctant to stand up for myself when Misty and Angus used bullying tactics, because I did not like my boring routine I was dispassionate about mainly because I was not doing activities I enjoyed doing. I let their bitterness destroy my confidence and self-composure. I felt down in the dumps when they made decisions for me. I cut myself off when they nagged and controlled me. They got the impression that I was being stubborn and difficult. I not had drawn to the Friday afternoon activities because I just was not interested. I did not enjoy afternoons out because I do things I do not like doing. I did not talk about my stress so I let the grass grow under my feet.

When my mum came to visit she offered to take me to the pub for a drink but I disinclined. She would not have told any body but I did not want her to know that I was drinking. I preferred to drink in secret.

In September ninety-ninety-seven I attended a therapy group ran by Brent and Hope. Tamsin, Wanda, Rodney, Kelly and Rico who later on dropped out We were chosen to be apart of it by Hope and Brent. Brent sprung it on us at six 0'clock *pm, the time the group* started. We did not have a choice if we wanted to go to it or not. I did not always like being apart of the personal development group. Some of the people especially Wanda repeated herself about her ex – husband and tormented childhood. I was not confident, sunny or affable. How I felt seemed frightening grew stronger every week. I took everything I heard with a pinch of salt as emotions were laid. I was not receptive to people unless I proved my worth. I did not want to be amongst the strugglers.

DARKENED LIGHT

We covered topics:

I need to break out of a rut.
I enjoyed being on my downward spiral so much I carried on drinking.
I have thoughts about fate, destiny mystical topics.
I do not feel sorry for my self, but I do sometimes sorrow brood and dwell because of the pain of loss time.
I see myself as a failure because my hopes collapsed. I think what might have been if I went to college at the age of sixteen.
I'm not grounded because I live inside my head.
When I fall a sleep, I wake up nothing is not there but a big emptiness.
I should try to look on the bright side of life
Stages of my life over the years have been hell on earth.
Sorrow, pain there is not a mountaintop insight.
I have inhibitions if it was not for bad genetics I would not be the inadequate person I am now.
I am inferior as well as inadequate.
To seek to gain is my motto.

I looked at the external world rather than inward. I wanted to make changes for the sake of a change. I opened up my mind in quite a big way. I am not always careful when making decisions because I listened to my instincts. In ninety-ninety-four, I did not take control of my destiny that would have led to a much batter life. I felt like a loser because of failures. Trouble times came calling. I should have been careful when that black cloud was over me. To get the full value of happiness I need somebody to share it with friends and find that place where I fit in and belong. I have not had much fun; I have not had romance, emotional fulfillment. I want to be apart of the outside world. Live day to day and have something to live for Angus talked to me about setting long-term goals for my self. He tried to persuade me to do worthwhile courses I was not interested in at a Training Centre. Wanda did a cookery course there but I was not interested. I was willing to get my life moving into a direction that would have got me somewhere. I am the only one who can take control of the next important stage in my life. I have to get out there and make things happen. I made it clear that it is not a question of if I start moving but when. Life is about constant change and movement. It is possible that aspects of my life and their accompanying problems were relevant to my stage of development. I intend to reach my ultimate destination, which is that mountaintop. I can see myself outgrowing Seven Wonders, the people there and moving 0n forward of my own accord. It was hard to know what is going to happen next. I do not find change unsettling or troubling because I am adaptable. I go with the flow and welcome a chance for growth and development. Play my cards right I will soon be looking smart.

I MADE MY OWN DECISION TO DO THE PRINCE'S TRUST

After I complete it, I hoped I would gain employment by going to college, and getting qualifications. I am interested in horticulture it is my first love and desire. I am aware whilst doing the Prince's Trust most of it will be hard graft. There will be times when I will wonder will it bring any kind of award. I will keep at it because I am persistent. I have the good intellect to achieve my hopes and dreams.

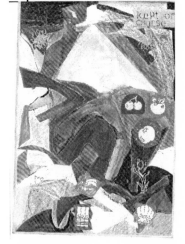

SUSAN SPLAINE

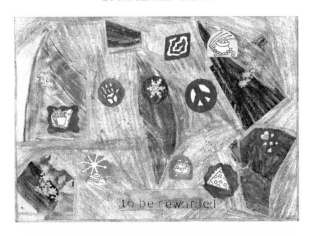

to be rewarded

CHAPTER EIGHT

I decided to do the Prince's Trust because I wanted to mix with people outside of Seven Wonders improve on my communication and social skills. I hoped to do a work placement something to do with horticulture. I needed the experience, gain confidence in my skills and abilities if I were to go to college. I needed to boost my spirits. Do something I could revel in; be enthusiastic about because for years, I was not aiming for any goals. What I wanted from the Prince's Trust was not clear-cut. I wanted to break out of my unduly routine. Time was passing me by I spent a considerable length of time in front of the television. I did not sit on the fence for very much longer. It was my aim to find satisfactory outlets, for both my personal needs and desires.

153

Monday February 23rd the first day of the course. Miles Cameron the team leader. Conrad Ashley assisted him. They are both a year younger than I am. Matt was the oldest member of the team only five days older than I am. I am ok at building up with relationships with people in authority I clicked with those two, initiated conversation because they have a sense *of* humor. Out of ten people, it was only Jay, Dean and I who were dedicated and committed to the team and intended to complete the three-month course people dropping out put the three of us in jeopardy. Other people had been on the course before but dropped out. They had another chance to do it again, but did not have a strong sense of duty, took days off. We did not pull together or work as a team. People sat in the corner and sulked because they did not want to be there.

I realized in order to succeed I did not have to stoop down to their level. I wanted to make progress because I felt it to be important. I started the day full of optimism, but not everybody appeared to help me remain a positive attitude. I had patience with them it was just a matter of hanging on until I come to the end; begin again on another three-month course. Too many different opinions resulted in chaos. They tested my patience, when I got annoyed with them; it was rather churlish of me because I gave into a stony silence. It was then when they offered me encouragement to do tasks and join in discussions.

SUSAN SPLAINE

When there was a stop and go feel about the day it was frustrating for me because I was all fired up and ready to go. I went with the flow and accepted not everything can be the way I wish. There was a tendency for me to float rather than keep my feet on the ground because I was bored. I played a supporting role because I did not want to let anybody down.

Miles had his own way of expressing himself when he praised me. The distance traveled does not count. It is the first step that is most important. I followed his advice and saw where a positive approach in life could take me. It was the first step of a journey into what it means to be the real me. I came to realize that sticking to the same routine and becoming stuck only goes backwards and not forwards.

I was not afraid to express myself to Miles because there was a great deal of harmony between us. I was envious of him because he talked in detail about his busy social life. I wanted to be apart of it because I was recluse even though I did not want to avoid social contact; under the circumstances I did not have a choice because I did not have anybody to go out with. Nobody in his or her right mind questioned the fact that I had come along way, but I still had some way to go to be more effective in social interaction.

The Prince's Trust is a twelve-week course. I did not complete it because people dropped out. It was doomed to fail on March 24 1998. The child within me did not want my relationship had with Miles to end. The next day my GP gave me antidepressants because I was in a nervous agitated state.

Four weeks we did:

We got together in groups of two and did team building tasks and problem solving, using mental agility communication and common sense. We went to the Fire Training Centre in Chorley. We did fire safety. The firefighter gave me guidelines what to do if I will ever become trapped inside a burning building. Keep fire doors shut. Open windows and say a little prayer. A Fireman did a demonstration putting out a chip pan fire. You put it out with a tea towel or fire blanket. You do not put water over it because it will engulf the room; sure to die because you will not have the chance to get out. On disused ovens, he lit some fires. Each team member had a go putting out with fire extinguishers.

On the residential at the Lake District, I did problem solving tasks everyday. We did abseiling and slept in a freezing cold cave. For the duration, we slept in something like a chattel. There was a kitchen in it, bedrooms with bunk beds in them. I slept on my own. A dining table, showers and toilets were facilities inside the chattel.

Community Project at Primary School in Darwen

We made mulch path. Dean made the sand pit by him self. I planted shrubs and made a rockery.

For years, I have felt I am lost in No-mans land!

The Prince's Trust was an opportunity for me to meet new people. Make room for growth with my communication and motivation. I was so fed up I could not get going because I did not have impetus to show a positive attitude make progress within myself so hidden capabilities will come out of the side to me that is repressed. In another six weeks, I decided to do the next course. I recharged my batteries so next time I could tackle it with an open mind. There was not anything happening in certain aspects of my life. I found myself thinking a great deal about matters that took place in the past.

I craved freedom, excitement adventure and variety.
I wanted success as a result using talent and energies
I was on the verge of getting onto a new open road.
I wanted to broaden my horizons.
I stepped out into the unknown.
I wanted a new beginning to happen in my life and a fresh start so that happy times might lie directly ahead.

News of Jasmine's baby Sid made me happy. Born on April 2l l998 I went to see him at her house a student social worker Lola took me, who was doing a placement at Seven Wonders. Paddy, Abbey and my mum were there. I paid them some attention they did not get snappy. I had my photograph taken holding Sid in my arms sat on a chair. He has curly blonde hair and blue eyes. Jasmine thinks he takes after her farther side of the family. Nothing to be proud off   All of us went out into Rochdale town centre saw Sidney working on the market. Sidney was high as a kite a proud father with nothing much to give.

On May 5, I did the Prince's Trust again with Adam Thurston I hoped this time round it will give me inspiration and make my life worthwhile; but I had to make the effort. I wanted many new doors to open and pave the way 'for the future. Make progress in ways that I never thought possible. I was in a chivvy to get my life into methodical order. I knew I was on the right track and success at my feet. To be confident of my actions the most important thing to remember; was not to move too fast too soon, after all timing makes the difference between success and. failure. There was nothing standing between me getting onto that new open road so that I could begin a completely new way of life. I could not change from being inadequate or inferior until certain changes began from within me.

I was ready to make my grand entrance on life's stage. I had every thing to gain and nothing to lose by pitching in and taking part in everything that was going on around me. I put others to shame with the way I knuckled down to whatever tasks we had to do. I can work in a team or left to my own devices. Two girls and two boys dropped out of the course. Everybody else was dedicated, committed and loyal and saw it through to the end. I did another Community Project at a school in Blackburn: Planting, painted a fence, made an archway out of logs.

A Fireman called Mick did First Aid with us all: Cardiopulmonary Resuscitation (CPR) is the first aid technique he taught us all. It is a technique used when breathing and heart rate ceases. It is a combination of mouth-to-mouth ventilation to restore a casualty's breathing, external compression to get the heart going again. Speed is vital, learn to feel for the carotid pulse and practice the positioning of body and hands, knowing when to stop is essential.

I practiced first aid on a dummy.
I checked to see if there is any danger.
Shake the casualty's shoulder.

There would have been no response if the person were unconscious.
Clear the airway: With the casualty's face upward, open the mouth and remove anything that is obvious with your fingers. Open the airway: Place one hand on the forehead and the fingers of the other hand under the chin. Press down on the forehead and lift the chin. This lifts the tongue to prevent it blocking the airway. I placed my ear close to the casualty's mouth and listened for signs of breath. At the same time, I looked along the casualty's chest and abdomen, for other signs of breathing. I checked for heartbeat: The only reliable way of establishing whether the heart is beating is to check the carotid pulse in the neck. I pinched the casualty's nostril took a deep breath and sealed my lips around the casualty's open mouth. I blew slowly and deeply into it to inflate the lungs. I saw the chest rise fully. I removed my lips and allowed the chest to fall fully then repeated the procedure. Check again for clear airway if chest does not rise. Give inflations at a rate of ten every minute that is about one every six seconds until the casualty can breath unaided. Get help somebody to send for an ambulance. Check the pulse after each time you have done ten inflations.

I did a practical exam: Cardiopulmonary Resuscitation, mouth-to-mouth ventilation. I also performed external chest compression. When heartbeat is lost doing first aid you locate the casualty's breastbone, which runs down the middle of the chest. Find the point at which the ribs meet in the centre. Measure two fingers width above this point, and put the heel of the free hand above the fingers, keeping them well clear of the ribs. Cover this hand with the heel of the other hand and tightly together. Kneel upright so that my arms are straight and move forward slightly so that my shoulders are directly above the casualty's breastbone. Then press down about 4.5cm. Release the pressure but do not remove my hands. Do fifteen compressions, counting one-and-two-and- three-and so on Do fifteen compressions per minute up to fifteen. This will result in a working rate of about 80.

I returned *to the casualty's* head, tilt the head back again to re-open the airway, and give two further breaths into the casualty's mouth. Give another fifteen compressions followed by two more breaths of mouth—to—mouth ventilation. Continue cycle of two inflations and fifteen compressions until the ambulance arrives. Check the pulse if the casualty's color improves: As soon as you feel the pulse, stop chest compressions. Continue giving mouth—to—mouth ventilation until breathing is restored then place the casualty in the recovery position. Check the heartbeat and respiration every three minutes to ensure that both are present. Be ready to re—start resuscitation if either of these vital signals should fail again.

<u>I did a second practical</u> exam with Mick: I played

the role of first aid. Mick the casualty cut his leg on a can of Lucozade. He fainted then fell to the ground. I raised his injured arm because it reduced the flow of blood to it. I controlled the bleeding by pressing a clean pad over his injured arm higher than the heart raised his cut arm. I raised his legs. He was bleeding heavily it would not stop. I continued trying to stop the flow of blood with continued firm pressure on the pad tightly over the cut. I did not remove the blood soaked bandage but applied another pad over the top of the bandage. The blood would not clot. I applied direct pressure by pressing a bandage over the wound. Urgent medical treatment the casualty needed urgent medical treatment. Waiting for medical help, I continued trying to stop the flow of blood that continued pressure. The patient went into shock it resulted from blood loss. I stayed with hum until the ambulance came.

Adam drove me to Blackburn Council because I had an appointment for the head of the parks department to interview me for my work placement in a greenhouse, situated in the parks department at a park in Blackburn. I felt nervous on my first day because I had never had any work experience. Two men called Ted worked in the greenhouse the charge hand was near retirement, the other one middle aged. Jade is younger in her thirties. Scott a sixteen year old also did a work experience.

Jade demonstrated to me how to pot plants. When

I had a go, it came natural to me so she left me unsupervised. I went out to the Council Office buildings with Jade. We watered the plants! We went to the Town Hall, Mayors Parlor and schools where we watered more plants. I had a bad headache because of my anxiety in the afternoon I was sick in the toilet, so Jade gave me a lift home. She had to stop the van because I was sick in the street. I took the next day off!

My work placement was for three weeks. I liked working in greenhouse as opposed to working in the gardens. I found watering the plants very relaxing. I did seed sowing, Propagation. I planted cuttings. I potted cuttings into smaller pots. I put pebbles into bigger plant pots just for decoration. Jade delivered plants to the army barracks in Preston to put on display for a party they had there. I made some hanging baskets and did' weeding.

I decided I wanted to go to Myerscough Agricultural College in Preston to study horticulture level 1 and 2 in September 98. There was nothing stopping me from rushing out into life. I was not frightened about breaking out into new directions; explore new avenues that could lead me to the pot of gold at the end the rainbow.

SUSAN SPLAINE

When the time comes to spread my wings, I must know where I am about to land. Any decisions that I make will have a lasting effect. I did what was best for me. I put my own interests first. I used what I have learned about other aspects of my personality to my advantage. I looked on the brighter side life. There is no limit to how much I can achieve and require once I redirect my energies, make the most of my talents. I moved fast and found the action stimulating. I kept it up to go with the flow until I have done what I had set out to do. I thought very carefully on matters that will change my life. I concentrated on my strengths not my weaknesses.

The final team challenge: We took disabled and special needs people out on day trips. We went to Knowsley Safari Park. Oswaldtwistle Mills. Watched Mouse Trap at the cinema in Preston then went bowling. We went to Camelot. We went to the Fire Training Centre. We raised the money doing a pub-crawl and a sponsored abseil previously on Friday. We did not do work placements on Fridays. We had a barbeque at the Prince's Trust office inside the YMCA building where there is a kitchen, and a garden. It saved money on a venue. Anti—depressants and calm tablets made me relaxed. I managed to mingle with some of the people. I do not like people liking me because I am charmed. I do not see myself as a magnetic person. If it was not for bad genetics, I would be magnetic. I have my faults and failings, but wherever I go I seem to be one of the favorites.

When we did the presentation, I was the only person who was not nervous because I felt at peace with myself. Firms/ companies who donated materials for the community project were invited. The people we worked with were invited nobody from the council came to see me. Hope, Brent, Kelly, Wanda and Rod came because we attended the therapy group together at Seven Wonders.

The venue **was in a bar in Blackburn** Town Centre. I drank vodka and coke in front of Hope and Brent. The Mayor presented our certificates.

Speech I did at the presentation about first aid:

By applying common sense and using the knowledge learnt on the training course, a first aide person can decide what treatment best in each case.
Assess the situation checking that the casualty is not in any danger. Make the area safe. Assess the level of injuries all casualties and decide treatment priorities. A first aide person can enlist the help of any bystanders controlling traffic or calling 999 for an ambulance, ensure that specialist help is on it s way. It is important for a first aide person to appear calm and take control of' the situation.
A first aide person will never approach a casualty unless it is safe to do so, never give the casualty

anything to eat, drink or smoke. It could make the victim vomit and could delay the administration of anesthetic. When deciding what is wrong with the casualty a first aide person must determine exactly what has wrong or how the accident happened.

Look at the casualty observing signs including breathing, bleeding and bruising. Listen to what the casualty and any bystanders say about the accident. Ask the casualty if any part of their body hurts, Smell the casualty breath and the around for gases, petrol and so on. Touch the casualty and gently examine the person for injuries.

What have I gained from the Prince's Trust?

I made my own decisions
A new door opened in my life
I got new ventures off the ground
I traveled in a different direction so that turning points will be ahead of me. I will know when I have reached the point in my life where. I wish to be myself, people to know me for my talents and not seen as a retarded person. I want to achieve a tremendous amount

CHAPTER NINE

Monday September 14 at Myerscough Agricultural College was the beginning of my horticulture NVQ Level **1 and two.**

Names of college tutors at Myerscough:

Basil Nekton: Course Manager. On Tuesdays, we did theory work with him. He also sometimes took plant identification classes.
Hazel Kendal did basic horticulture with the students.
 With Jason Beverley, we did plant identification, written tests and turf.
Titus Frond did landscape.
Gawain Wilkin did machinery.
Ned Bland did glasshouse work.
Reynolds Cornell did glasshouse work.
Caradoc Tapping did tree nursery.
Jeremy Blair did ground care.
Percy Manley did soft landscape.
Julian Beamy worked on the golf course.

Every Friday I got 1OO percentage in plant identification tests. I did landscape practical tests such as Fencing, flagging and building a wall. We had to get full marks in written tests to pass the course. My vegetable plot also went towards final mark.

SUSAN SPLAINE

Topics NVQ Schemes:

Safe lifting, fencing, health & Safety, plant Identification, planting, turf from seed, fire safety, line
Marking, pruning, First Aid, Chemical Spillage, Paving, Machinery, Vegetable Plots, Garden Design,
Pest and Disease, Safe use of Tools and Machinery, Propagation and tree care.

Searching for new paths, I found inner peace and happiness. I improved my life by making a dream a reality. I made up for lost chances. What I know about myself now, I could put to profitable use in the future. I had more confidence than I knew what to do with. I thought about where I am heading! Making a success of my college course, I hoped it would lead to a horticultural job. Success tasted so much sweeter for me because I know how it feels not to achieve anything.

I made the most of my appearance, smiling happily at the right people. I have splendid determination to do well. I made the most of my time. All that I needed was a bit of enthusiasm. Other students were sunny, bright and humorous. I found all the cooperation I needed whilst working in the glasshouses. All I had been asking when felt unsure if I was doing something right or wrong. I did not think that it was a sign of weakness. I needed a helping hand from time to time. I was patient with those who were less intelligent than I was. Outside working all day, it turned out to be a little more hectic than I thought. I had lots of work to do. I tried not to over do it. I aimed my sights as high as possible. I showed my gratitude to those who supported me. I used my instincts because they told me new faces that are worthwhile.

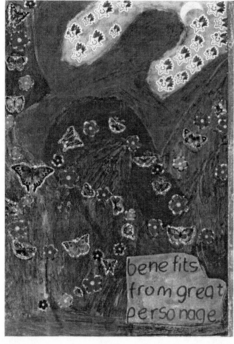

I lived in at college in October ninety-ninety-eight the next day Hilda and Benjamin came to visit me. They were overjoyed and pleased for me. They mentioned to me about the next step to move to Webster Street. In my review meeting, Benjamin always said people cannot live at Seven Wonders forever but can get very comfortable. I was aware of the fact that Hilda and Benjamin made the decision the time as come to move out of Seven Wonders and live independently at Webster Street. Hilda and Benjamin had a meeting with, the staff at Seven Wonders planned out the next year of my life. Go back to college to do a much more advance course that does exams. Then move into my own flat. At that point, in my life I just wanted to get through college. After it finished I was not sure, what I wanted, or where I was going. I did not plan that far. I had always been negative about Webster Street. I did not want to move there. It is a cheap terraced house with cheap second hand furniture in it. It was impractical because there is only one kitchen. The three other residents take turns making meals with a staff member. I will make my own because I am vegetarian. I will not be able to make my meals until after they have eaten and washed up. There was not enough cupboard space for my cutlery and utensils.

On Friday, I went back to Seven Wonders for the weekend. Monday morning Ezekiel drove me to college. On Tuesday evening, I still went to the Personal Development Group. Oscar picked me up after college, so I could attend it on time at six thirty in the evening. On Wednesday morning, I had to get up at six thirty, caught the early bus to Preston. From there I caught the bus that took students to college. Angus took leave from Seven Wonders to go to University in Manchester so Brent took over being my key worker. On Friday nights, he worked at Final Resting Place. Brent also lived there in a little flat that is in the old people's home. I went to see him every Friday evening at seven 0'clock for an hour for counseling sessions. I also drew some pictures.

Pippa my roommate moved in a week after I did. She studied Agriculture NVQ Level 2. She was the only girl on her course just as I was the only girl on my course. I managed to build up a good relationship with her. I found it easy to communicate because something clicked. I often kept my own counsel where possible will only use one word rather than an entire sentence. I wanted to know what she was feeling and thinking. Pippa found my interest in her flattering relationships therefore were well starred. She was eighteen going on nineteen in November. On my course, Sean was the oldest in his thirties. The other lads were aged 16-19. The age gaps did not bother me. I got on well with some of the students.

Pippa was always in a sprightly, fun loving and inventive frame of mind. Pippa is good natured I trusted in her because I am listless. At night, she had her male friends in the room she knew from the year before when she did the foundation course thick people do. I did not have much time to myself because the room was always crowded. I resented being tied down to places, conditions and faces when I did not enjoy it. I am too loyal and peaceful! I did not tell her that I need more space and emotional freedom I have had of late.

They all came into watch my television and videos people brought in. I picked and chose my words because I treaded very carefully, where the sensibilities and feelings of others were concerned. I did not want people making judgments because their perceptions can be wrong. I was in the right frame of mind to let my talents lead me into a new way of life. She occasionally went out to somebody's room so I was able to relax and have a quiet moment.

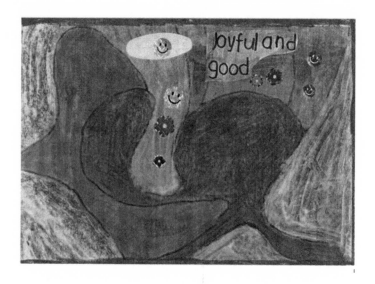

I went to the gym most evenings after my meal. I went to the local pub on my own when I felt like a drink. I sometimes went into the college bar with Pippa. Doing college work passed the evening by quickly. On Monday morning when I received the test sheet to revise plant identification, I knew all ten plants by Monday night. The tutor taking plant identification classes told students the names of the ten plants, taught the common and Latin names. The tutor taking the lesson put all ten plants into the library where we could go to learn them. When we did the tests on Friday morning, the plants were numbered and laid down in the classroom on tables. With my numbered test sheet wrote down the common and Latin names. I could not always sleep at night because I felt hungry. Pippa brought her own cold drinks, coffee, milk, sugar and snacks, crisps and biscuits. I could only afford to buy my own coffee, milk and sugar. I felt like a trashy tramp because I did not have any money.

I was on the road to learning knowledge about horticulture, which in turn would make room for growth. I saw the path ahead much more clearly, because my book was not my only ambition. Usually I plodded along in life, for reasons best known to myself there was a certain urgency to get things done. During the day, there was a lively feel about it. I thought twice about taking on heavier loads. I enjoyed working in the glasshouses.

Working days ran smoothly for me and the other students. The tutors were always in a humorous frame of mind. It helped the day to pass quickly as well as productively. I fulfilled my obligations without overdoing it. I could cope with college work because I had high expectations of myself. I had the confidence, became adventurous and light-hearted. I charged through with the work I had to do. I found fencing and lawn mowing two of the most boring subjects. I did not like working on the golf course, so instead I worked in the glasshouses. I am not a green Keeper! I took to path work, flagging, planting and pruning. It is in my nature to be a good horticulturist. I would like to work in the parks department or in a greenhouse.

In November ninety-ninety-eight Rojo and Hope, told me that it is time I should move into a dump of a house. I do not need to be at Seven Wonders anymore because I am at college. I do not need that level of care. Apart of me did want to move to get away from Rojo. Since I have been there, she has not stopped looking at me maliciously. Rojo and Hope had the idea fixed into their heads for me to move. I was not very effective with them because I would not have changed their mind. I agreed just to please them, because it was what they wanted. I let them know by packing my belongings into boxes in December.

It hyped up that I would like it in the house on Webster Street, because at weekends we go out in the afternoon. Everybody was up for me moving out. I did not make my unhappiness known to Brent, because I expected him, and Hope would sing sorrowful tunes to me because they thought that I pity myself. Whenever I did not agree with them, they told me that I am being negative. I felt full of doom and gloom... miserable about my impending move.

Social workers moved me into Local Authority Housing because I could not find the right access to the right kind of help, and support at the time I needed it. It was vital that I moved out because I could not grow or live with deadbeats. I had problems because of lack of help and information. I needed to know what help to seek. I had difficulty getting employment because I did not go to college and even employers whenever I did go for job interviews perceived me as a retard. Living with deadbeats did hinder rather than further my recovery. The chance came to move so I took it.

I did not want to move to Webster Street. I had many ideas inside my head how to escape. Write a letter to social workers or run away. Over Christmas, I felt physically ill. I was in a glum mood. Family members did not come to visit me. I treated myself to some new clothes. Nobody were not sure when two Lovers Wanda and Rodney, were going to move out of Webster Street. I felt anxious a waiting my time for them to move out. In March ninety-ninety-nine, Wanda and Rod moved into the same neighborhood as Webster Street. Rico and I moved in with Ramon and Josh. I new deep down that I would find away out. Clinging onto hope gave me the courage to see it through that I would get out of Webster Street. On Saturday, Brent helped me transport my belongings in his car. I did not have to unpack in the kitchen because boxes I packed with my kitchen utensils in them I used as my cupboard space. Some pictures and ornaments I kept in boxes on top of the wardrobe. I usually adapt to new surroundings, but I did not there. Jeremiah and Tukishi were support workers there. She gave me a lift to college on Monday mornings.

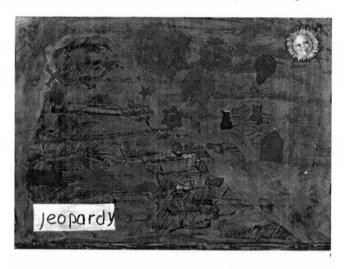

jeopardy

I accepted that it was the wrong path for me because I did not fit in. I did not talk about my unhappiness. I thought a lot about how much I hate life. Jeremiah made sordid comments that he found me attractive. He would always make comments about me in. front of the other residents. I felt uncomfortable and embarrassed that he got pleasure from it because I made him laugh. He drooled and stared at me. I took his compliments as an insult. I felt like he wronged me! I felt ashamed to tell anybody because I do not think much of myself. He joined the cause behind all the other sordid men his age who, lusted after me. I am not a man's fantasy you see in strip clubs. What he saw must be somebody who has innocence and purity about her; they should not judge people from what they see on the outside. I see myself as a dark cold person who is not in a good mood for very long.

If I did report him, I would not have been able to cope with the aftermath, all the displeasure and tension. Talking does not always resolve problems or life's situations. I could not face up to a confrontation with him in the same room with Hope, Rojo, Ezekiel and maybe Brent. I could not bear to be anywhere, near him. I felt hopeless because I could not find away from making him stop treating me the way he did.

I dreaded the Easter Holidays having to stay inside that house for three weeks. I was in a dreamy state. I kept my mind focused on how I am going to get out that house. My anxiety level was high and I had depressed physical symptoms. It was a reaction to how Jeremiah was treating me. At college, I felt like I do not want to get out of bed in the morning because I could not face the day. I sometimes stayed in bed instead of going to lessons. I lacked interest in college work because I could not enjoy it anymore, because of feelings of sadness. I felt distracted inside my own mind because of my slow thinking. There was a decline in my physical strength. I could not get to sleep at night. I did not enjoy the company of other people because I cut myself off. I started drinking a lot again. All I could see were grey skies and black clouds. I decided to write a letter to Hilda and Benjamin. I hoped they would get me out before college finished. Break me free from the hurt and pain. There will be sunshine after the rain. That black cloud will shift and fluffy white clouds will appear. To feel better and find inner peace and happiness my life situation needed to change.

On March, 21 my dad's sister Sadie who I never see came to Webster Street at six 0'clock in the evening with Hope and my two sisters. I knew it was a flying visit they have some bad news. The bad news is my dad is dead! He went on a barge boat to Norfolk on his own. During the night, he fell into the cold rigid water. The shock killed him. He actually did not drown because he was wearing a life jacket. Ernie's passing did not have an affect on me. I did not feel a sense of loss! Sadie said she would be in touch to tell me when the funeral is. I thought to myself what funeral. It had not registered so I told her I am not going. It was my decision to make. Nobody had control over me. It felt, great. I went back to Seven Wonders with everybody in Hope's car. Those three did not come into the building with me; they went straight back to Sale in Sadie's car. I spent four days sleeping in Sandy's room in my sleeping bag. I would not lie down on my back because dead corpses lie down on their back. I kept thinking of him getting up in the middle of the night falling overboard trying to do a reconstruction inside my mind. I could not feel any sad emotions. I would not go out on my own because I felt numb and fragile. The day seemed to drag because I did not know what to do with myself. I talked Sandy into doing the Prince's Trust I even went to the office with her to get onto the next course within a few weeks.

I wanted to see my mum over the phone I arranged for Rory to pick me up in Blackburn. My mum's eyes were puffed up and red. She cried for somebody she did not love, who meant nothing to her. He brought her nothing but misery. I felt compelled to give her a hug, physical affection and words of comfort. She had plans to move to Rochdale to be close to Jasmine. Ernie has left her behind life insurance. She is planning to spend it on a new house, move to Rochdale to be close to Jasmine and Sid. Jasmine stayed in Sale with Sid and her Jack Russell dog, Bingo. Abbey has a spare bed in her room, so both of them slept in it. I felt agitated inside the house because it was just so harrowing and scary. I would not go upstairs on my own to get my stuff that had been there since I moved. I had box with all my diaries in it for my book. I wrote it all into textbooks before I moved to Seven Wonders. I took my treadmill back to Webster Street with me. Rory drove me back with Jasmine.

My mum shouted aloud to herself through out my childhood because she had no money; it made her feel miserable. It was a desire of hers to have money. She regretted having kids because she thought she would be better of money wise. Every month she will get Ernie's pension from his work place. I wanted to do a memorial: Draw a picture of what I think heaven looks like. Write a goodbye letter and bury it underneath a shrub I want to buy and plant in the garden at Webster Street.

On Friday April 9, I went out looking around Blackburn Town Centre. An Asian lad called Mazola, who is my age chatted me up. He first asked me if I have a boyfriend. He invited me to go to the pub with him, to have a couple drinks so we could arrange a date and get it together. I told Mazola about all my life's troubles as I do to complete strangers. I arranged to go out clubbing with him then go for a curry. I gave him my address and phone number because he wanted to pick me up in a taxi I phoned up Brent at Final Resting Place told him I could not make it to our counseling session because I am going out with Pippa. It was a believable story because she knew couple of lads who lived in Blackburn. During our social event, I was prepared to communicate with Mazola by telling him lie after lie, just to make a good impression and lead him on.

We went to three pubs in Blackburn. He could not

get into the club because he was wearing jeans. We went to Accrington in a taxi, Mazola's hometown. At the club, he is a regular. I drank different drinks at the club in Accrington. Mazola drank either coke or lager. He seemed proud to have me on his arm. He had a broad smile on his face. At the curry restaurant near the club, the waiters knew his name, so he must be a regular in there as well as the club. He would not stop smiling or looking pleased with him self. It made me feel uncomfortable. He walked me to the house where he lived fortunately for me he could not get in because when he put the key in the keyhole the door would not open. He shouted up to somebody to let him in, but the person living there would not get out of bed. He tried kissing me on the doorstep. I was not up for it so he took me to the taxi office and came back to Webster Street with me. He arranged to see me tomorrow. He phoned but I would not go out with him. I gave the impression that I am easy going. I was hypersensitive because I wanted him to buy me drinks.

I do not find it flattering because men just want me for one thing. If I were a prostitute or worked in brothel men would not want me. If a man did want me, passion and chemistry would not be there between us. My thinking and behaviour has not changed over the years. Behaving as I do does not boost my self-esteem. It does not boost my self-confidence. If I tell the staff at Seven Wonders about Mazola, they would think that I make myself vulnerable.

On Sunday April 11, I arranged to meet Sidney outside Blackburn *Market* so I *could* go to his house spend the night there. On April 12, I wanted to attend Ernie's funeral. He went out to play squash then he went to the pub. I stayed in with Jasmine and Sid watched the music channels. I did not like today's music any more because I missed George. I found it intolerable listening to the radio. I hated manufactured bands and singers because George cannot compete against them. If he sings songs that are deep and meaningful, make people cry his records will get to number one. I hate songs singers singing about feeling lonely without their partner. Love of their life becomes their life their whole world. A person in a relationship likes to have time to him or her. A partner does not become your life, your whole world if your life is not empty. I could not tolerate Sidney when he came back drunk at 8.00 pm. He stroked my face with his hands and looked at me with admiration. I think Jasmine could do without Sid if he ever goes to a clinic treatment for alcohol abuse. She will not have a longing to be with him, because she does not love him.

Sidney's sister Patty looked after Sid because Jasmine did not want to take him to the funeral. He drove the three of us to my mum's house in his beat down, banger of a car. My mum's two sisters and brother in-laws were already there, so was her brother. My mum waited with anticipation for the Hearst to come. She just wanted to get on with her life and spend her money; move to Rochdale. When the Hearst came, I got into it with my mum, two sisters and two brothers. We were not a family in mourning. Sidney drove in his own car to the graveyard. My mum's *family* drove in the same car. Ernie's two brothers and sister were at the graveyard when we had all ready arrived.

It was an outdoors' service on a cold, wet, damp, gloomy day. *Work* colleagues were there to pay their last respects. The people at the funeral meant nothing to him. He was content not having contact with his own family. My eyes did well up when Abbey and my mum cried. My mum, two brothers and sisters have adopted his self-centered attitude. In *times* of sorrow, we do not help each other or pull together.

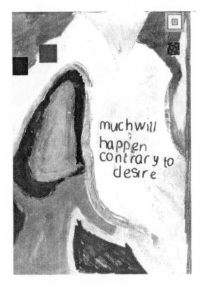

much will
happen
contrary to
desire

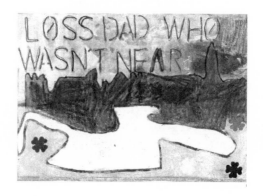

I went to my mum's, house in the Hearst with my family. I felt scared inside the house because I had a sense it was spooky because of his spirit. We did not get together as a family to have a wake for him. He has gone forever I will not miss Ernie I do not think his parents brothers or sister will not mourn him. Sidney and Jasmine gave me a lift back to their house, so that I could get my stuff. I caught the train back to Blackburn I felt vulnerable on my own because I wanted comfort and tenderness. Tukishi and Jeremiah offered me their support if I needed to talk. I can go to them whenever I want to. I had a bad headache I just wanted to go to bed. I could smell Ernie's body odor in the corner of my bedroom. I would not move the chair because I thought Ernie's spirit was on the chair. Mazola phoned me up on that same night. I arranged to meet him in town the next day to tell him he is not the love of my life.

I did not have any contact with my family. I did not

bother making contact with them by phone, because Jasmine, Paddy and my mum only main concern was Ernie's life insurance. On April 19, I went back to college. I felt sad emotions. I felt tearful and had weeping fits. I did not always respond when people spoke to me. I hated it when people asked me did you have a good Easter. I will not ever have a good Easter until I reach the very top of my mountain. I did not feel the need to talk about Ernie because we did not have any form of a relationship.

Life is precious nobody knows when it is your time to exit the world. Life is a journey on a wide-open road. When it is always raining I felt like I am not going anywhere fast. I do not feel happy with life for very long. I do not get the blues because of bad memories. I did not feel hopeful today, yesterday or tomorrow. To feel good about myself I need to find that elusive kingdom where I fit in and belong.

In May, I went on holiday to Oasis with Brent and Misty, the three residents who lived at Webster Street. Jess who used to live at Webster Street came along on holiday with us all. Toby, Willa and Paul from Seven Wonders, also went on holiday. Ezekiel drove us there in a mini bus he hired out. We rented two apartments next door to each other.

I shared a bedroom with Willa. At night, I could not relax or get to sleep. When I am not being very sociable Misty and Brent, get very disappointed with me. They also kept on saying how well I am doing because I was coming to the end of my College Course. I put on an act that I was in a good mood for every body's sake. I did not want to be as much fun as a wet blanket. I felt like I was under tremendous pressure because Misty and Brent expected too much of me. I went on the roller blades with the other people. We ate meals together in the same apartment. I went to the Cinema with Misty and Willa. We watched you have mail. Everybody else watched Shakespeare in love. We went on bike rides and went to the disco at night. We all watched a musical on our last night.

Brent and Misty did not realize that I was drunk on one occasion because I was being chatty. Deep down inside I felt sad and was hurting. I walked around on my own because I wanted peace and solitude. In one of the pubs, I saw a woman order lager with blackcurrant; it became one of my favorite drinks. I could not get enough of it. It was as if I was becoming addictive to my new topple I got pleasure from it; because I needed more too drink. I drank to cope with the misery I felt. I was also confused because I could not understand if I was happy or sad. I do not think I did not want to be happy because happiness is the color of the sunset. I could not workout if my clouds were cloudy or blue. I hated spending too much time on my own. I do not want to live a life of loneliness and solitude.

On Wednesday June 9, I felt like I could not carry on with college work. I had completely shut down. I could not find the words to describe how I felt. I went back to Webster Street: told them I have caught a bug going round. I felt even more fed up being back there. I felt like ripping my brains, and banging my head against a brick wall. I felt agitated and angry but I do not understand what made me angry. If I expressed my anger, I think that I will probably have seizures and convulsions.

Minor problems needed changing before they got bigger. In the pub over a pint *of* lager and Blackcurrant, I wrote a letter to Hilda and Benjamin. I wanted that black cloud to lift from over me. Jeremiah irritated the life out of me because of my intolerance. I found his behaviour overbearing. It seemed like the right moment to act. I had a belief they would get me out of there. I spent over £300 on my credit card it arrived in the post on the same day I went on holiday. I brought new clothes, compact discs, food and alcohol. I did not think it was time I cut back on items I did not need, because it was not often I treated myself. Money problems do not create stress for me. I went to the bank to see Magnus, the accountant who was dealing with my money that was in an interest account. I told him that I want to close down the account. He told me there is an escape clause. He made an appointment for me to go and see him on Friday. I did not go to my counseling session with Brent because I went to the pub instead. I could not face him singing sorrowful tunes to me as he always did whenever I was unhappy. I reached that point I stopped expressing myself to him. I did not expect him to phone because he did not run around after me.

On Sunday, there was an open day at college. I told Tukishi I am going to help. I was not going to, really, I just used it as an excuse brought alcohol bread and salad and biscuits. I paid by credit card. I put the food and alcohol inside a cooler box in my bedroom. I had to go out for pub lunch even though I did not want anything to eat. I sat there at the table, whilst everybody else was eating. We have to go out on the activities because all that matters to the staff at Seven Wonders is it is the taking part that counts, it does not matter if you will feel fed-up going out with them. At college, I was glad of some peace and solitude. I had the room to myself because Pippa was at home. I shaved the sides of my hair with razors, whilst the grand final of stars in your eyes was on television. I swept up the hairs on the floor with a hairbrush. Ian Moore won the contest, he sang woman in red. It was ironic because an old male friend told me that red is my colour. I drank alcohol for my breakfast. I went out to look around the stalls. People made comments about my hair because it looked a mess. I behaved in such away that expressed sad emotions. I did nothing to help myself because I was not good company.

When Pippa came back to college on Monday, she was worried about me. She kept on fussing, telling me to talk to her, why I cut my hair. I could not find the words to express how I felt. On Monday morning, I went to my first lesson. When I went to my room, Zoë the caretaker was cleaning my room because Eli my cleaner was on holiday. I started crying she asked me "what is the matter". The first thought that came to mind was *my* dad has died I did not even know myself why I was crying. Zoë told me that it is the shock. She took me to Sherry's office she deals with the

residential side to the college. Zoë explained to her why I was upset. Sherry phoned up the doctor so she could prescribe with anti-depressants. The doctors made an appointment to go to the surgery on Wednesday. I felt overwhelmed by their affection. I did not know how to cope with the strong feelings of despair.

SUSAN SPLAINE

I was lawn mowing when Benjamin phoned me up at college. The office worker in Basil's office came to see me. She had the phone number of social workers workplace he gave it to her so she could phone him back I just told him that I want out of there. Hilda and Benjamin came to see me on Thursday afternoon they met me outside the college library. They drove me to the local pub. When I tried talking to them, they interrupted me and ended my sentences. Nothing I said or did was right. I did not have a say what I wanted to do with my life. I felt stuck and deformed because I was not making my own decisions. Hilda threatened to put me in a bed-sit if I do not comply with her. Rot away inside my black hole without any support. I gathered they are not going to move me out of that house. I let them bully me into a situation I did not want to be in because I did not want to stay at Webster Street. I felt tied down and pushed into a corner. I did not plan to play into their hands. I had thoughts about running away after college finished. I told them I would somebody to stay with they took it the wrong way, thought I meant one of my tutors. I did not have to shout and scream to stand my ground to escape.

I believed that I would triumph my own way and feel pleased with myself. I decided the best option is to keep a big distance between us; do not turn to them again, it was possible under the circumstances. I decided to stand aloof from fighting with them or with anybody else at Seven

Wonders. I was determined to be my own person with my own mind and action of behaviour. I did not want to be the trapped person Hilda and Benjamin wanted me to be. My unhappiness did not depend on those two treating me like a puppet on a string. I was in a progressive frame of mind to make my world a much better place. I would not let anybody tighten their grip on me, because I could make my own decisions. What mattered to me the most is I wanted more independence and personal freedom to do as I please; nobody to answer to because people in authority can be controlling and take over by making decisions I do not want them to make for me. Rules and regulations were less likely to get in the way of my search for space.

Brent phoned me up at college to inform me that Hilda and Benjamin told him I have been drinking. Rojo and Oscar wanted to see me at three 0' clocks late afternoon I felt betrayed Benjamin phoning up leaving me to face those three on my own. Where is the support in that? Living at Webster Street made me feel ill and messed up nobody did not recognize that fact. I did not care they wanted to see me. I did not have the resources to go because I expected Rojo would give me a telling off as she always did whenever I was in their wrong books. Instead, I went to the bank to see Magnus. I needed some documents that were at Seven Wonders. I shouted at him demanded that he should phone Ezekiel. I let off Steam slowly. I kept my mind focused on getting my money, then getting out that house. I went to bed at five 0'clock in the evening because of all the upset and I felt dizzy. I dreaded going back to that house after college finished. I could not avoid Jeremiah in the house because he is intrusive. I could not talk to anybody about him because I was not on speaking terms with anybody. I was thinking negative when I wrote Hilda and Benjamin a letter. I should have known they would not get me away from the hurt and pain.

I had the right to complain! I did not do it to make people angry with me. I could not understand why everybody was giving me the cold shoulder, because of my black period. Therapist could not see past my ugly behaviour so they could not see my pain. As the day went on my mood did not improve. I blamed myself because of the emotional state of desperation and frustration. I blamed myself for being such a weak person because I am capable of being much stronger because I have good coping skills.

On Monday morning June 2, Jeremiah and Tukishi drove me to Seven Wonders. Rojo and Hope wanted to have a showdown with me in a small-darkened room. Rojo sat dead close to me on the small two seating-sofa fuming. Hope in front of the door so I could not escape. Jeremiah sat down on a chair he would not take his eyes off me, neither would anybody else. Tukishi on the floor used the wall as a backrest. Jeremiah stared at me for so long without foaming or drooling because he was too annoyed with me. The encounter I had with them was very intense. I gained some piercing insight into when I am illogical in my behaviour it makes them tick.

They were hard to cope with. Everybody was seething. Hope was always in deep thought. Rojo's eyes penetrated; her face angry and red. She had her finger pointed in my direction, tried to make eye contact with me because my eyes I was looking blankly at the wall and not at her. When Hope thought of something to say about my past life events, she laughed and had a dirty smirk on her face, mentioned my double rape, the time when I fell into the canal because I was not sure if I fell. I will end up dead because somebody murdered me. She mentioned Alex. He is a brief encounter I let pass me by because we did not get it together. I might have a nervous breakdown because of it. People who do not find happiness do breakdown when they think of loss chances. It was horrible Rojo tormenting and being dead close to me... She would not stop raising her voice at me. She took a breather when Hope interrupted being sly and sarcastic. She mentioned the time when I met up with two American Mormons. The time when I went to Sale for Christmas on the same day my mum told me to piss off so I got into a taxi back to Blackburn. I got it from Salford because it is only a straight road passed Bolton.

Both of them wanted to know what I brought with

my £14 allowance. They thought that I did not eat meals at college because I brought food to snack on when I felt hungry. The portions were only small and a piece of fruit afterwards. She thought three meals a day should be enough. I was very active during the daytime. During the evening went to the gym, it speeded up my metabolism. After five thirty in the evening Rojo thinks it is forbidden to eat I have to wait until breakfast.

I went shopping with my credit card because I was biding my time until I get my money. Rojo thought that I should be deprived having anything new. People with low self-esteem do not treat themselves to luxuries, so mine must not of been that low. I rebelled because I did not let her drag me down to her and Ezekiel level. I do not like cheap food or cheap clothes. I have my pride and standards. My high standards traits I get it from my mums Auntie June who was a snob. My mum's sister Freya also has high standards. I might come from a trashy immediate family, but I do not want to be a tramp!

Rojo took my anti-depressants off me: She told me that I am just sad. I was very tearful and crying. I showed signs going back to old behaviour I was trying to change my ways. Support workers did nothing to help to get me out of my psychological rut. When people spoke to me, I spoke in riddles. Hope and Rojo were much more annoyed with me because I did not make any sense. My mind was full of fog. Hope told me how much she is angry with me. I was angry too and it was not just, because controlling behavior makes me tick.

On Wednesday June 3, I went back to college for the last two days. I was under orders from Rojo and Hope to write an apology letter to Benjamin and Hilda. Pippa was glad to see me back because she missed my company. I sorted out my portfolio folder. I was not bothered because nobody came to my presentation on the last day. Collecting my certificates on stage, I was gloomy. The old people who lived at Final Resting Place were due home from their holiday in Blackpool. Ezekiel passing through picked me up in the mini bus. I did not know what to think in the van with just the elderly.

When he dropped them off at home, he took me to Seven Wonders. The atmosphere was too tense because of stony Hope. She did not even speak to me or acknowledge that I was there. A negative thing he did taking me there. When he drove me to Webster Street, I did not even unpack. I went to the local pub, drank couple of pints of lager with blackcurrant.

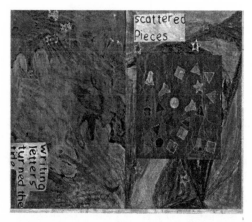

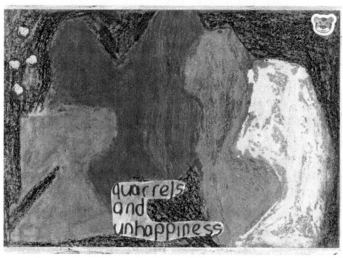

DARKENED LIGHT

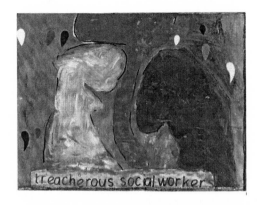

treacherous social worker

CHAPTER TEN

I felt as if I was at a turning point in my life. There was not anything I could do but wait for a new direction to appear right before my eyes. My despair drove me to confide in social workers. I had the right to complain, but it put me at considerable risk. I festered about a showdown I had with four very bitter and hostile people, because I wanted a vicissitude to take place, I was not ardent about living inside that house. Rojo and Hope accused me of being **a** wrongdoer. It is ironic Rojo saying she gave me security. She had always been sly with me because of her stone-cold stares. All of my tension and inner frustration it came from somewhere. I felt I needed to let rip, let out my aggression I felt towards her.

Every Monday morning Rojo went to Webster

Street, gave Jeremiah money to give to us; she also had a meeting with Tukishi and Jeremiah about the running of the house. She gave me dirty looks, so I stayed, in my bedroom just so I could avoid her. When the residents spoke to me, I was slow at responding because it was too much of an effort to communicate because of my distrait mind.

Jeremiah threatened to tell Rojo if I did not enjoy myself on the weekend activities, because I did not snap out of my glum mood. I did not pretend I was having a fun time because I did not want him to give her a false report. I let Rojo and Hope - disturb my peace of mind. Life became unduly difficult, led to me not being on speaking terms with them Hope, I have not ever been on I and Rojo only usually spoke whenever she gave me a telling off. However much I was hurting I was still encouraged to spend time in the company of others. I dreaded going to Seven Wonders so I could take part in the Friday afternoon activities. Rojo looked at me maliciously. Hope was always snappy with me. The tone in her voice was one of despise. She would not do a programmed with me even though she kept on saying I need structure during the day. Other staff members gave me a mixed reception. I found them overbearing because of their intolerance. I suffered from the feeling everybody were against me. I lacked support because they felt offended because I felt like I came to the end of the road.

DARKENED LIGHT

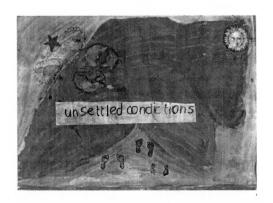

unsettled condictions

My life came to a standstill because my time was not satisfied. I stopped going to Seven Wonders to visit Sandy at weekends, and during the week. I was aloof for my own reasons distant, reserved and standoffish. I felt rejected by everybody I felt scared and lonely. I did not have anybody to turn to during my darkest moments because I was feeling black. I found time for peace and solitude in my bedroom at night because I felt tired and edgy. There was a big distance between myself and other people; to the extent, I could no longer see them. I had a vision in my mind I am in a tunnel escaping. When I looked back Hope and Rojo were smaller and smaller. In my review meeting, Hilda and Benjamin were very controlling and dominating. They did problem-solving exercises with me; why are Rojo and Hope so angry with me and disappointed. I could not find a logical solution to make the situation better. Nothing I said was right! I went with the flow! There were not blue skies overhead because I was not out of the woods.

It was partly because of how Jeremiah treated me I built up a brick wall. I wanted new doors to open. I noticed Jeremiah was annoyed with me because of my miserable mood. He stopped drooling over me because my black emotions rubbed off onto him. I felt like banging my head against a brick wall and pulling my hair out. How he was with me, I used it as the excuse to run away. Pent-up emotions needed releasing. I felt like I was dying inside that house when stuck in because I was not motivated to go out so slept in the afternoons. I spent my time walking around aimlessly in the evening because I had much more energy. My life became unbelievably complicated. I finished feeling bruised, bleeding and frustrated. I coped with lost tempers because of annoyed professional people. Money matters were not on my mind but on Ezekiel's. He fretted about the state of my bank balance. He insisted on going to the bank with me, so he could watch me sign on a dotted line I had no intention of fulfilling, leaving my money tied up in a long term interest account.

I want a father figure that is why I like older men. If I belonged to a different family my dad would have meant the world to me. My mum never loved me. He was never there. She never held me. He never cared. Growing up alone I never had a hand. I tried to hold on forever to find my own way.

DARKENED LIGHT

On Tuesday July 6 at around 6.00 pm, I walked past a Hostel on St. Peter's Street; men with psychiatric problems live there. Robbie shouted out of his window: "hello". He asked me to wait for him. He is a tall man aged twenty-nine. I liked him because he is rugged and rough round the edges. –He also had a sense of humour. He came out of the building smiling and making direct eye contact at me. I felt child like and wanted somebody to cling onto a friend was with him, he did not have enough money to go back home to Preston on the train. We went to the train station with him; he went on a train without paying. Robbie invited himself round to Webster Street for a cup of coffee. I told him I live with four men but he did not find it off putting. I was very trusting of him because he lifted my mood. Robbie was very comforting because he listened to me as I talked to him so I allowed myself to get intimate with him. I thought meeting him was something meant to be. He had just come out of hospital because he had a nervous breakdown. He also had a 'tormented childhood His dad used to hit him with a belt.

When we got to the house, I took him upstairs to the bedroom. The other residents were in the room next to the kitchen' listening to the radio. They did not see him come in with me, but probably wondered why I had two cups of coffee. When Jeremiah came at l0.00 pm to give the medication I told him that I am going to bed so do not disturb me. Richard tried kissing me but I did not want anything sexual to happen between us.

He wanted to go home; he did not go because I wanted him to spend the night. We slept together in my bed. - I had a need for physical contact and warmth because of Hope and Rojo's- aggressive behaviour towards me. The next morning Ramon saw him leave. He promised not to tell anybody. On Friday, I told Brent about my new relationship with Robbie. I thought I did the right thing being open and honest. I did not worry too much because I was not taking life seriously enough and it caused me problems.

I went through some unpleasant confrontations with Rojo, Hope and Ezekiel. Rojo told me to forget about feeling tired because I am bored and not sleeping. Hope asked me how much I would charge if I were a prostitute. I took it as an insult because I wont' put myself in a position where a man will force him self on me ever again. Hope insinuating that I behave like a prostitute. They were all annoyed with me, could not decide what to do with me because of dilly-dally. I made a hasty judgment meeting Robbie. They asked me if I had sex with him, also I am a great looking girl. I do not think I am. What I see is a person who looks like a man. If I were a man, I think I would look like David from the X Files. He is attractive so if I were a man I might be much better looking.

They told me not to go out on my own and to stay in. I had to sit at Seven Wonders bored during the day. I battled through; I did not let frayed tempers get the better of me. I still saw Robbie a few more times. He came round to the house when Rico was in they greeted each other by shaking hands. He fell asleep because before hand he smoked dope. I went out shopping on my own even though there was a new rule I cannot go out by myself. I went to the gym. I went ice-skating. I went out on my walkabouts and to pubs.

A big change in a person's personality and behaviour is the first sign that something is wrong. Physical weakness, doom and gloom were not short-lived. I did not get any guidance or support. I wrote another letter to social workers because of problems encountered.

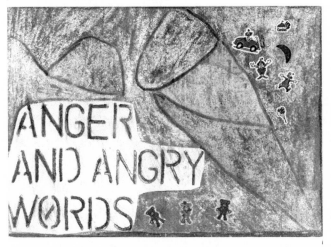

July 30 Ezekiel moved me back into Seven Wonders, into my old flat. Willa who I went to Oasis with was living in the same flat. Carmen was still there. On that same afternoon, I

barricaded myself in my bedroom at Webster Street. I put my bookcase in front of the door. I did not want to go out on the Friday afternoon activity because I am a coward. It meant going to Seven Wonders. Rojo and Hope giving stone-cold looks. Ezekiel came round to the house; threatened to phone the police if I did not remove the bookcase. He managed to persuade me to open the door. He was calm and patient as opposed to raising his voice, as he had been doing since I finished college. He told me that I am not in a fit state to go back to college, put it on hold until next term. I wanted to spit in his face when he said we are tying to help you. I had not seen a friendly face over the past three months. He talked me into going out because I needed to be in social situations.

At Seven wonders I went into the house, Hope gave a stone cold look so I stormed out of the building. She came after me because I ruffled her feathers, because she had a lot of anger directed at me. She raised her voice and said, "How there you ignore me" I reached the point I just found it amusing. I can take abuse because I learnt in childhood how to cut myself off from upheavals and bitterness. I hated everybody because relationships were not good. I just walked away. Ezekiel and Tukishi came after me in his car. I got into the car even though he was furious with me. Nobody could not see past my ugly behaviour to see that I was also angry despairing. I could not understand why I was feeling the way I did. He was right about one thing it was my intention to put my placement there in Jeopardy, because I did not want to be there anymore.

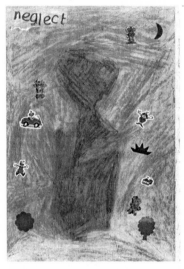

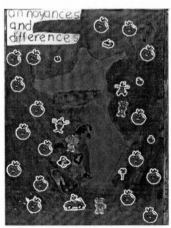

Life was grey and unexciting. It seemed like the

rain would never stop. I had to stand a lone. They turned my world into circles. I needed somewhere to run to because I wanted to get away from Seven Wonders and Webster Street. I needed somebody who would make me laugh and cry at the same time because of heated tensions, and bad feelings. I did not bother drying my tears when I felt upset. I just let the tears flow because when I did cry I would just suddenly stop then cry again. I needed a shoulder and a caring, voice. On Saturday, I felt less tense because Rojo and Hope were not around. In a very sensitive state, I imagined the worse. It is easy to focus on the cloud rather than the unseen benefit.

On Sunday, I went back to Webster Street because I could not face Hope or Rojo the next day. Jeremiah phoned Rojo, told her that I am back there. I just wanted to have laughing fits when she said, "if I can not face people it means I am not feeling safe". She was annoyed with me because of her and Hope's resentment, just because I wrote a letter to Hilda and Benjamin expressing my unhappiness. She was under the impression I needed staff around me to cause me more misery. I wanted to get as far away from them as possible. I went to bed at 5.30 pm because I felt tired because of mental strain. I did not go downstairs to the morning meeting because I felt edgy. At 10.00 am. Hope came into my room. She behaved as if everything was rosy between us. It was like old times. She was being smiley, nice and pleasant. I hated her for not recognizing that she and Rojo had pushed me to the brink of despair. I was in a dark horrible place. I needed to find my way back. She told me that I am unsettled. I need to go and see my GP. I could not go on my own because I needed her permission. It was important for me to make decisions, to introduce significant changes in my life.

I could not take the strain or tolerate living there anymore. I was tired people taking over my life and deciding what is best for me. They spoke to me as if I was back for the long-term. Misty asked me every day if I am looking forward to going college. When am I going to get my stuff back from Webster Street I just thought to myself somehow I will get out of here. On August 3, Hope went with me to see my GP. She diagnosed me suffering from depression. I felt strong feelings of resentment towards Rojo; she told me that I am just sad. I did not talk about my trouble times with the doctor. I pretended I felt the way I did because my dad died, just to keep the peace. I did not have the strength to face more showdowns and discussions. She did not have any knowledge how bad it was there. She prescribed me with anti-depressants; suggested that I should stay at Seven Wonders for three months, and then move back to Webster Street.

Hilda and Benjamin came to see me. Had a meeting about the direction my life is going in with Hope, Ezekiel and Brent. They took me to a cafe in town, brought me a horrible jacket potato with salad that made my mouth dry. Once again, they kept on interrupting and ending my sentences. They were only concerned about — why was everybody angry with me. Benjamin said, "It is all locked up inside your head". Hilda made up excuses but could not find answers to my predicament because she was very bitter. They were very disappointed because I hated it there. Every body's only concern was if I am going back to college. They wanted to have another meeting to make the final decision if I am going back to college. I had thoughts about doing what I did to get out my mum's house. I was tempted to take an overdose of pain killers outside the hospital then tell a doctor.

I still was not on speaking terms with anybody. My behaviour was such a rush it carried them away because they did not know how to deal with me appropriately. It was the end of relationships with them. I had the desire to be free from constraints and restrictive lifestyle. I could no longer cling on to that area of life. I was being kind to myself because it was unlikely anyone else were. Days had been wretched. The mealy-mouth attitude of certain people did not help. I tried not to make the matter worse by overreacting or imagine I did something wrong. I knew deep down that I was not the cause of that atmosphere. I wanted to retreat from the fray.

I went to the bank on my own to get my money.

DARKENED LIGHT

On the computer system, Abbey's name and address came up where she lived with my mum in Rochdale. I told Magnus to write down the address for me. I made the decision moving to my mum's house is my escape route. I took advantage of Ernie's death. If he were still alive, I would not have turned to my mum. I listened to my instincts telling me the time has come to change direction. I was confident that I could make a difference to my life. Feel at my best with changes I want to make. New doors will open if I take one-step at a time. It was time I pushed myself forward of my own accord. I wrote another letter to Hilda and Benjamin. In it, I mentioned that I have discharged myself from Seven Wonders. I wrote down Jasmine's address and phone number, because I did not know my mum's address or phone number. I decided to leave quietly and post it when I get to my mum's house.

On August 13 Ezekiel decided that he wanted to go to the bank with me so he could put my money into an interest account. I did not want to tie up my money. I agreed with everything he wanted me to do because I had enough displeasure. It would have made him tick if I disagreed. I made the decision Friday 13th is my leaving date. My loss will be a blessing in guise.

I told everybody "I'm going to Jasmine's house this weekend for a break". It was all right by them, they let me go. I phoned up Jasmine told her that I want to visit our mum. I got my haircut because it was a mess. I treated Sandy to a night out at the cinema. We watched Star Wars. I was determined to have fun and spread a little happiness On Friday morning I went out to Accrington on the activity with Misty, Noreen and Kane. Instead of going out in one big group, one staff member took three or four people. I felt so excited I could not stop talking because I found away out of Seven Wonders.

Ezekiel drove me to the bank in the afternoon I left my bags in the trunk of the car because he also wanted to give me a lift to the train station. He let me have £6OO to last me all year. He put £3000 into an interest account. He drove me to the train station helped me with my two bags. He stayed with me for about 20 minutes until the train came, brought me a cold drink from the cafe. He could not help himself but mention if I am going back to college. It was an option. I kept my mind focused on escaping from "hell on earth". I am not moving to paradise but it will be a fresh start and a new beginning.

DARKENED LIGHT

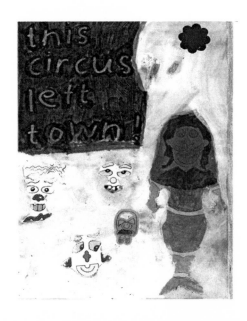

When I got onto the train to Manchester Victoria, I felt as if a big weight had lifted of my shoulders. All of the tension I felt gradually withered away. I caught another train from Manchester to Rochdale. I caught a taxi to my mum's house. Sid was there with her because on Saturdays Jasmine works as a security guard in Bury Car Park. Abbey, Paddy, Jasmine and Sidney were out in a restaurant. Zandra is happy now that Ernie is dead but she has not mellowed down. She told me that she is all right for money, because she gets £300 pound every month from Ernie's workplace. I told her I have moved from Blackburn. She was fine about me staying with her. It is only a three-bedroom house, so I had to sleep in the lounge in my sleeping bag. She was not curious why I ran away. I posted the letter I wrote to Hilda and Benjamin.

I established a strong rapport with my family they placed a big demand on my attention. I lived at the house until I find somewhere else to live. I did not expect everything to happen all at once. I was confident I would get my life into methodical order. I will mature, grow and flourish. I was sure of myself that life will become more enjoyable, pleasures and thrills. The potential was there to bring out my true self in any way I wanted to.

Hilda phoned Jasmine, she gave her my mum's phone number. She arranged to visit me on August 24. Hilda and Benjamin did not want to listen to my side of the story. My expectations were too high in the first place. Hilda was a bitter cow! She seemed too had dipped her tongue in vitriol, judging by her apparent determination to find fault with everything I did. Tried to put me down by telling me I am not streetwise. Why I make myself vulnerable is the dark side to me nobody knows about. Sometimes I feel like I am becoming somebody else. It is my true nature thinking or behaving the way I do Hilda thinks I have not moved on or changed. She was unsure what my needs are. I did not want her to appoint me another social worker, because social workers take over your life and want to be dominating when it comes to making decisions that is best for you. Hilda also wanted to know what I spent £500 on I did not tell her because she thinks like Rojo I cannot have any new clothes or com pact discs. I paid of my credit card bill and brought new clothes. She raised her voice before and after our encounter.

Benjamin made witty remarks. He thought I was not ready to work. When am I ready to work? Is he going to get in contact and let me know! I did not want to stay in waiting for his elusive phone call that was never going to happen. He said I am dependent on the council to give me a flat. If they do not give me one, I will end up on the streets homeless. If those two were not working as part of a mental health, team I would not of gotten a placement at Seven Wonders. They moved me in there and expected the staff to bring out my true nature. There are two sides to a person's personality but I still cannot describe myself as a person. When Hilda and Benjamin became involved in my troubled life, I was standing at a crossroads. I waited for a light of hope to shine down on me.

Abbey phoned up a removal firm. The removal men arranged for me to go to Blackburn on August 25 so I could get my belongings. I felt like I could not face every body without alcohol in my system. Alcohol was like a friend I became dependent on drinking to face hostile people at Seven Wonders. I had thoughts they will all revile. First thing in the morning, I drank lager and blackcurrant in the house. An hour before the removal man was due to pick me up at 9.30 pm.

In a flask, I drank coke and Martini. A young man called Cameo picked me up in a transit van. He was so polite. I drank alcohol in the van out of the flask on our way to Blackburn. I found Cameo easy to talk to so I was very talkative. Conversation seemed to be non-stop. I think I talked a lot because I felt hyperactive, so we did not have uncomfortable moments of silence.

We went to Webster Street first but nobody was not in at home I felt disheartened because of it meant going back there after I have been to Seven Wonders. We decided to go to the bank so I could withdraw £50 and pay him for his services. On our way to Seven Wonders, I did not feel scared or nervous, because I felt so happy. Brent greeted us at the door acknowledged us in a particular way. By the look on his face, he was festering because I made my own decision to move. I did not let him intimidate me. Benjamin told me everyone was shocked because Rojo and Hope did not see it coming. They did not register the fact that they drove me away just because I wrote a letter. Carmen and Willla were not inside the flat. I did not see anybody else. Brent waited outside whilst I cleared out the room where I used to sleep. I left a box on the wardrobe so it meant going back. Brent once again greeted us. As I was leaving, he asked me if I want to say goodbye to anybody. Cameo was aware of the tension it made him feel uncomfortable. I told him we fell out. Ramon was in at Webster Street all by him self. I took some plastic boxes with me but all of my stuff was in black bin bags. Ramon helped Cameo and I to load up the van. On our way back to Rochdale, I was still talkative. It did not take long for us to unload all my bags and boxes into the house I paid him £70 and gave a £4 tip. He was very grateful brought his dinner with it. All my stuff that was in bin bags I put them into boxes. I put boxes in a storage cupboard, in Abbey's bedroom, in my mum's bedroom and in the lounge. When she buys a new house, most of the stuff will go into the attic.

After a few days, I did not feel good or contented with my lot. I felt much more emotional because of strife and discord. My mum and Jasmine told me to stay on the sick. Do nothing with my life. I felt insecure because I am an outsider, but I did appreciate she let me stay with her. I kept my cool and kept calm so all will be well. I wanted harmony instead of quarrel. Paddy told my mum that I was drunk when I was not. She would tell me to stop drinking. I told her I had not been drinking. It was like a mad house because of Paddy and my mum. Outburst every day shouted at each other. Abbey joined in. That black cloud had not drifted from over them. I do not think it ever will. If I shouted back, it would have caused long-term damage. She would have said hurtful things to me. It is not easy talking to Zandra when she is in one of her bad moods. I just ignored her by not saying anything. I did not know how many nights I could take before I got hot under the collar. It was very uncomfortable sleeping on the floor in sleeping bag.

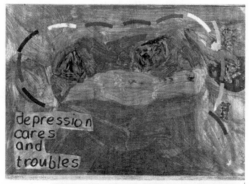

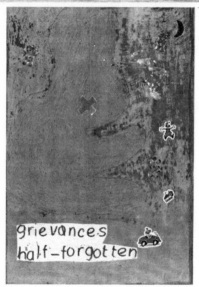

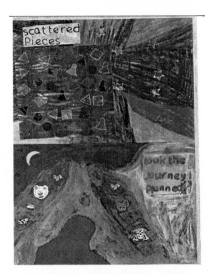

CHAPTER ELEVEN

An unpleasant period in my life ended. I wanted to start functioning properly again. It was my aim to open new doors. I am able to map out a lot because of my ability to take the long-view, work out exactly what I need to do to get out of my black hole. On Monday 13 September 1999, I went to see a career Adviser, Roy told me about the New Deal Environment Task Force. I wanted to do the landscape course at Groundwork in Oldham. He gave me some information about eligibility. I was eligible to enter on the New Deal within three months because I have been in Local Authority Care. I made an appointment to see a Claimant Adviser so that I could sign on to jobseekers allowance.

Within three months, my life moved into the fast lane. I knew deep down I chose the right path because I am particularly creative in what I do. I was not always in a rush because I slowed down to a more comfortable rate. I will gain a great deal by cooperating with people who can help me reach my mountaintop. I spoke to Cindy at the housing department she did not want me to move into a flat on my own. She decided that I should move into supported accommodation because I had just come out of care. I hoped she would say that! I did not want to live in a flat on a rough council estate. She suggested that I should go to the homeless office across the road. I spoke to Danny he offered me immediate advice and gave information on my housing difficulties.

He wanted to know why I moved from Blackburn. I told him the story then he took down the address where I lived, my mum's phone number. I looked in my phone book because I do not learn numbers. He saw the number of social workers in my book, he wrote it down because he wanted to speak to them to get some details about me. I wanted staidness and conformity in my life. I wanted to rearrange my time how I occupied it to prevent myself feeling claustrophobic. I did not want to feel smothered because of entrapment.

DARKENED LIGHT

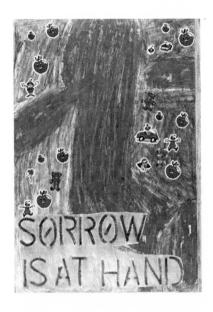

Abbey, Paddy and my mum are couch potatoes. I watched programs I did not usually watch. Abbey would not let me sit in her bedroom so I could listen to music and handwrite my book. I sat on the stairs until everybody went to bed at about 10.30 pm. Paddy, Abbey and my mum do not stay awake until late. I wonder if sleep can be genetic. In the evening, we went out for a curry once a week. Abbey babysat Sid because she has gone off curry. When Sid slept over on Fridays and Saturdays, he brightened up the evening. He slept in the spare bed in Abbey's bedroom. Sid is restless and energetic. I devoted time to him by playing with his toys, reading books and playing with Lego. I built up a rapport with Sid within a few weeks. I felt close to him in return he felt close to me. We bonded together.

My mum still got up at 6.00 am every morning. She put the Mountain dog, Bruce into the garden every morning. She shouted at him. She would not give him time to have a stretch before she got hold of his collar and dragged him up. I went upstairs into her bedroom with my sleeping bag. I went back to sleep on the floor. I hated mornings because the television was always on. Paddy talked babyish to his mum. Kept on saying will you be posh when you move into your posh new house. I think I tolerated him much more when he was shouting. I could not wait to move out so I could have peace and quiet in the mornings. I went out on my walking around aimlessly just to get some peace. I took an A to Z with me so that I could find my bearings. Abbey did not always answer me when I spoke to her. She was not always my favorite company. On some day's she was a lot more bearable. Relationships were difficult to handle when everybody were at each other's throats.

Every two weeks on Mondays I went to the job centre to sign on I also had a discussion with Sally my Adviser about job search, even though I was a waiting my time to do the New Deal. I wanted the opportunity to meet mew people. I enjoy spreading my wings. On October 26, she arranged for me to join a job club. I hated the idea of waiting to get on to the training course. It felt like the right time for making things happen and getting instant results. My approach to life is practical eventually however long it takes usually achieve my aims. I hoped for the positive aspect and the pot of gold at the end of the rainbow. My goals were realistic.

On October 27, my mum moved house. The street where she lives now is near where tramps live so she has not moved on from humble beginnings. I moved into the dining room where I slept on the sofa. Paddy still talked babyish living in a nice house. I had a bad headache at the job club. Holly who worked there told me to take a few days off. Mae a member at the job club asked me if I wanted to go with her, when she does voluntary work with the British Trust Conservation Volunteers.

On Sunday, I arranged to meet her outside the pub, near my mum's house. At 9.45am, the team leader picked us both up in a van outside the Town Hall because that is the pick up point. I introduced myself too Gary the team leader. Opal was a volunteer team leader. Three men and two Women were the other volunteers sat in the back. We went to Sholver in Oldham to meet up with the Ranger, Sheridan. We spent the day planting Oak, Common Ash and Alder Trees. I felt self-satisfied doing an activity I enjoyed doing. I like the cold weather and the wind blowing against me. I got on with Mae had conversations with her and other people.

Abbey is pregnant her baby is due in February next year. She is not in a relationship with the father of the child. She will be a single mum living with our mum and big fat, piece of nothing Paddy. I hoped I would be out of there before the birth. I longed to live in a much more peaceful household. At the job club looking for jobs in the Observer, on November 2 I saw a job advertised for a support worker in supported accommodation in Castleton. I wrote a letter to enquire if they have any vacant flats if I can move in because of my circumstances. I saw it as good luck falling down from the sky into my lap. I see a dark side to me nobody do not see because I come across being vulnerable. I have astute and shrewd characteristics. I seek to gain in that sense I will not stay stuck. I think if a criminal mastermind taught me how to be a con artist I will be good at it. I do not show remorse or guilt so I could carry on as normal, look victims in the eye.

I reached the end of my tether sleeping on the sofa bed. I felt remote and cut off from my family. I felt inadequate but not beaten by circumstances. It was easy to mope, but it was more productive and rewarding to channel my energies into activities that brought me satisfaction and comfort. I did not appreciate my mum and Jasmine bossing me about telling me not to do nothing with myself, stay at the house forever because it is comfortable. The more they tried to hold me back, stand in my way the more rebellious and bloody-minded I felt. I pity Paddy because he has not matured or developed his personality. He still has temper tantrums and violent outbursts. It is not hard for me to accept I am the 'black Sheep' of the family. I will not ever be in a highly emotional state affected by it. On November 6, I received letter reply back from Shelter. Tilly the manager was not available to see me because she was off work. She will get back in contact with me.

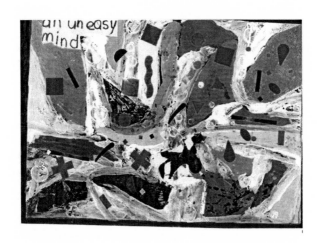

On November 8, Sally arranged for me to have a Mentor. Lynn from the Tameside Education Business Partnership came to see me at the job centre. I needed the kindness of professional relationships to touch me deeply. Not all of my feelings are comfortable. I was not confronting emotions I considered ugly, unworthy of myself. It is far better to face up to them, let go than hope they will mysteriously disappear of their own accord because they will not.

On Monday November 15, I got a letter back from Shelter I had an appointment to go for an interview on November 19. Jasmine, Paddy, and my mum came with me to make sure it is not a dump. I did not want them to come into the interview with me so they waited outside in the garden. There are sixteen flats with one bedroom, lounge and bathroom. There are ground floor flats and second floor flats. Jasmine approved that it a nice enough for me to move in I had my interview with Tilly the project manager, and Melba a key worker. I felt fantastic in the meeting because I was able to defend my corner without trending on anybody's toes. They wanted to know how I got myself in the situation I found myself. Two heads were better than one. Tilly will make good judgment on me when she makes the decision I can move into Shelter. The decision made to move in based on good judgment. From pain, I gain by putting misery behind me. I deserved to feel pleased with myself because I was in a realistic and practical frame of mind it helped me to act in my own best interest. Tilly informed me she will have a meeting with the staff there because I referred myself the staff had to make a joint decision.

On Monday 29 November, I started my course with Groundwork. At the induction, three other lads were also there, because they are doing something else that is on offer. Building work, decorating and office work. We filled in forms with Margo about rules and regulations. I had the opportunity for learning, growth and potential. I follow my hunches and feelings rather than relying too much on common sense. I was on a new open road. In the far distance, I saw the mountaintop that is still miles out of sight. My good luck stars shining through. I stood underneath my light of hope. I want happy future, success, contentment and joy.

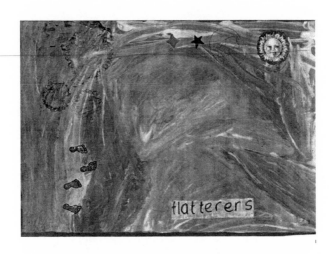

SUSAN SPLAINE

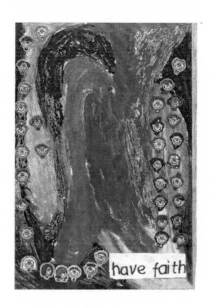

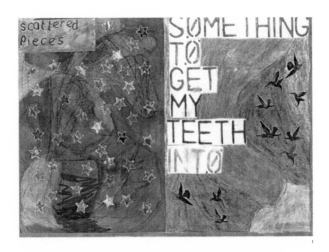

CHAPTER TWELVE

On my first day, I *missed the* bus that went straight to the Groundwork Centre in Oldham. I had to go in a taxi so that I could get there on time, it cost me £8. Jack my team leader was off sick. I worked with Duke another team leader. I also worked with another Jack who is on my team. Duke picked his team up outside the Town Hall in Rochdale because he had a task to do, doing up a Council Estate in Rochdale. There were four boys working with him, a student Patsy who was studying Conservation at Hopwood Hall College in Middleton. We did planting and mulching a pathway on the surrounding fields. For a council estate the ambience and landscape is delightful. I was committed and dedicated because I liked the work, got satisfaction from it. I am dependable and responsible. Occasionally I was relied onto such an extent. I was somebody Duke could rely upon because the other workers felt fed-up and could not be bothered.

Every morning I got up at six thirty from the bus stop outside my mum's house, I caught the bus into Rochdale; from there I caught the bus at seven forty five to Oldham. It took about forty minutes to get there because there were school kids at every bus stop a long the way, the traffic busy. When I started work with Jack, he depended on me and the other Jack for our loyalty, reliability. Mark was forced onto the course by the job centre he did not have a keen interest in the work. He did not want to be there he took the odd day off. He never did a full attendance! It was the planting season: We planted bulbs near woodlands in Stake Hill. We planted a rose hedgerow at a nursery in New hey.

A woman from the housing office at Rochdale Council phoned me up told me she has made an appointment for me to see a Duty Officer at Town Head Social Services. I needed a social worker to be able to move into Shelter. Despite the falling out, I had with everybody at Seven Wonders, Hilda and Benjamin I did not lose faith or stop trusting people in authority. I did have exaggerating worrying thoughts he would ask me questions, why I ran away. I did not intend to get into fights and arguments. I have my faults and so do them. Nobody showed me love so I did not get rid of my bad ways. I have never felt guilty about taking advantage of Ernie's death. He did nothing for me whilst he was alive. Ernie dying made great headway so I could head for the hills. Will anybody care because I have real cause of complaint against him because my feelings of hatred are genuine?

I went to the pub an hour before my appointment to see the Duty Officer. When I got to Town Head Social Services, he did not want to know. I did not need to see him because I do not have a psychiatrist or a social worker. I felt despondent because of anxiety I might not move into supportive accommodation I believed in myself that I
would come up with ideas that would dispel negative thoughts. There was not really much point in trying to talk to him because social services can be a lot like Mickey Mouse Circus. The decisions I made, my views should be pivotal. It might only be a matter of time before everything slots into place. That man phoned up Tilly at Shelter so she could talk to me on the phone then he wondered off somewhere. He was not the least bit interested. I felt stranded. Tilly wanted to talk to Hilda and Benjamin at their office.

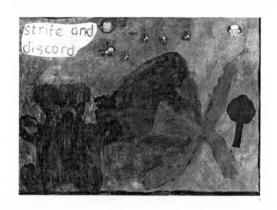

I did not feel positive about the outcome of their phone conversation. I didn't want Tilly to tangle with Hilda her thinking is as rigid, as her ideas are incorrect about me, because she thinks nothing is not wrong with me, I do not need support I was ready to back up my statements even though she will never agree with me. I was sure she would say things about me that will be heartfelt because of bitterness, she felt deeply about my behaviour. She will make it sound sincere what she thinks about me, put pay to me ever moving out my mum's house.

Every Thursday it was college day at the Groundwork Centre. I should gain NVQ in Environment Practical Skills. Pearl a bossy woman took us for our lessons. Greg was a volunteer who helped. He had a sense of humour I clicked with him. I had a portfolio folder I put my written work in for safekeeping. I answered questions on handouts about Health & Safety. Greg is knowledgeable about the scientific side to horticulture. He helped me to answer the questions on handouts about trees. In the afternoon, we went out, did what they called field studies. Local residents used a field as a dumpsite. I was confident answering questions and discussing the covering topic.

My spirits lifted because there was a lively feel about the day. On wet rainy days, I did not complain because I did not want to sit in the van until it stopped raining. On most days, people I worked with were busy and rushed off feet because there was so much to do. I was capable showing Jack I am bright, knew what I was doing. He left me to work on my own initiative because I did not need him watching over me. I was not always staid because I let Mark when he turned up push me onto the sidelines, so I did not shine through. I waited until Jack told me what to do. I enjoyed being out in the fresh air. It is my fuel, gives me energy.

My weakness was fencing because I am not very good at hammering nails in. I did not mind digging that was the easy part for me. Jack was coming to the end of his course. An assessor called Wade came out to site to assess him a few times. Whenever he did, I pressurized myself because I felt I had to prove myself to him, but he did not acknowledge me. I hate it when I think people think that I am disinclined. I do not let criticisms or people looking down their noses at me dent my confidence. I progressed, my skills. I could see hidden capabilities coming out.

I have a behavioral problem writing letters when I want to enlist help! I wrote a letter to Sheridan who I met working with the British Trust Conservation Volunteers. I had escapist encounters from the realities of life. I expected him to let me do a work placement with him, let me stay in a cottage near his workplace; support me into making my world much brighter instead of dull. When I worked with him, again tree felling he said that he had received my letter, with a grin on his face because he thought it was amusing. He told me that somebody is starting a work placement with him. I behave like a buffoon because of my impulsive, reckless behaviour. I never realistically wanted to work there or move into a cottage. I was in a dreamy state confusing my instincts with illogical thoughts. I wrote that letter in a fit of a pique. I lost contact with Mae because she stopped going out with the British Trust. On Tuesday December 21, we had a barbeque outside in the office garden on a cold winter's day. People were talking and laughing. I felt as if my mood was going down. I felt so far removed from everybody and found it a strain making contact.

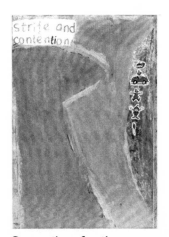

Strife and contention.

Over the festive season, I had the flu spent all week in my mum's bed during the day. Jasmine, Sidney and Sid were there most of the time. The tension and strains were beginning to show when my mum shouted because I was ill. I looked tearful, miserable and unhappy. It was not so long ago she kept on shouting at me because she thought I was drunk when I was not. She shouted out to everybody I do not know what is wrong with her. Then she will have a moan aloud to herself. She got frustrated because I was not feeling all right

What do I want to aim in the year two thousand?

Carry on doing my course with Groundwork.
Move out of my mum's house before February that is when the
Baby is due.
Build myself up and develop my skills.

Life is a gift what I do with it is my choice.
I want my mood to alter when the picture changes to how I want it.
I only want to feel happy when I have something to be happy about in life.
I want my life to move at my own pace.
There are changes a plenty on the way as I will soon discover.

On January 5, I had an appointment for a Mental Health Support worker to come visit me at home about moving into Shelter I felt downhearted because she did not turn up. During discussions, if people listen to me I find it easy to express myself. The more open-minded and optimistic I can be, the more I will benefit. I want the decisions I make to have a lasting effect. I want to do what is best for me, put my own interests first. I want promising days to bring new challenges to my life. Explore new horizons and find comfort. I hoped for the positive aspect and the pot of gold at the end of the rainbow. On January 7, I listened to my instincts telling to take the day off because my life is going into a new direction. I received a letter from Shelter I can move in on January 10. Moving will benefit me in the end. My family was trying to tighten their grip on me, not to move but stay at my mum's house. My mood felt much lighter than it had been. I was feeling bogged down, flat and strained.

I went to MFI, put £35 deposit down for a storage unit to put in the lounge. I hoped my mum would lend me £306 to pay for it. I pushed myself into a corner because I felt restricted and hampered. Paddy did not approve because he is as much fun as a wet blanket. He poured cold water over my suggestion when I told my mum by giving into a stony silence. He did not need to say anything because our mum did not care what he thought. She willingly wanted to help me out. Despite being in the grip of some intense emotions, he helped bring down my stuff from the attic that was in boxes. I put it all into boxes in the garage ready for the removal men to load the van the next day. It does not take me time to get used to any major alternations.

Two removal men helped me transport my stuff to Shelter. I did not find it too stress full or hectic because I have good organizational skills. Miriam a Project Worker gave me the key to my flat. The two men unloaded my possessions, whilst I paid my £5 deposit for the key I paid £6.05p rent, filled in a housing benefit form. It took me a couple hours to unpack my clothes, cutlery and put my books onto the bookcase A lot of stuff were still in boxes until my storage shelf unit is delivered a week on Friday. Miriam gave me a lift to Tesco down the road because I needed some food: she also told me to get my electric card from the local garage. I will have to go there when I need to top up my electric. I had a good nights sleep in my own bed for the first time in months. Melba was my key worker at Shelter. She is the oldest staff member there. She is caring and easy to talk to person. I took the day off from groundwork to wait in for my shelf unit.

I did not go to college on Wednesdays because I thought I was going to Hopwood Hall to do NVQ Level 3. I was waiting for a date to attend an interview so I could get onto the course one day **a** week. I received a warning letter in the post because of my time off. I had a fear about confrontation with Oona and Margo; they deal with the timesheets and administration. I had fantasies inside my head they would torment me. How I thought and perceived what would happen in reality did not. I told the two of them I thought I did not have to go in *on* college day. I have a vision inside my head I am on a stage show before people confront about my behaviour. When I have had a showdown, the curtains come down. When I went for the interview at college, I did not want to do it because level 3 is about Management. On Wednesdays, I went back to college at the centre. I always seemed to be in a good mood because I liked the theory work, I got on with Greg. The more sociable I am the better I like it. I get on well with people with a sense of humour. Vic another instructor did conservation and plant identification with us.

DARKENED LIGHT

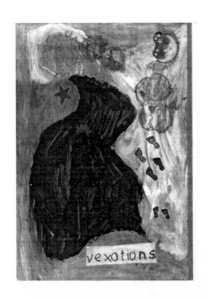

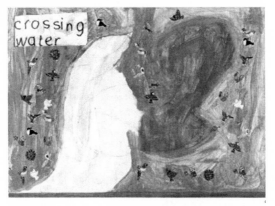

SUSAN SPLAINE

Jack still worked with Jack as a volunteer: He finished of his fencing. Two new lads started on my team. Kent and Byron were committed and dependable. They both had good practical skills. Mark still did the odd day, so did Lex. We did conservation work with Jack. We also did hedge lying at Stake Hill in Middleton. We did a boardwalk at Boar Shaw Clough. I liked to work on my own initiative because it passed the day by quickly; even on wet damp, rainy days. When the clouds are grey, it makes the days go slow and take up my energies. I slogged away to try to make time pass quickly. I found mulching around trees, planting very relaxing jobs.

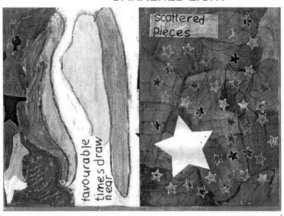

scattered pieces

favourable times draw near

CHAPTER THIRTEEN

Duke's team will be working on the housing estate for a long time because there is a lot of work to do. Haydn's team worked on a housing estate in Oldham. The people on those teams, if they want to can move onto (ILM) Immediate Lab our Force after three months come off job seekers, get paid £109 a week stay on the course for another nine months.

On January 21, I started work on Duke's team: Blake was on the Immediate Lab our Force. Andrew was coming to the end of his six months on Environment Task Force did not want to do Immediate Lab our Force. The other lads just turned up when they felt like it. A girl named Ada, who was a volunteer she liked to take centre stage, be in the limelight. I did not have much to do all day because there were too many people. When Ada was not, there I did her jobs. I let her push me onto the sidelines. She had a very good working relationship with Duke, so he always made sure she had work to do. Blake was always miserable I did not speak to him he did not talk to me. Andrew did not say anything to me or to anybody else in the few weeks I knew him.

For months we planted trees, shrubs, did mulching on the surrounding grassland. We also did fencing, litter picking and seed sowing. I was not able to show that I was a valuable member of the team. There were problems with Duke's power complex because of his urge to give four lads and Ada all the jobs to do. I did not like it because it was vindictive but I was unable to retaliate. I felt tense, overwrought and rather grumpy. Sometimes there was a rather subdued atmosphere. I thought Duke and Ada were being hard-face. I did not assert myself because of lack of confidence on my part, or the stern attitude of Duke and Ada. I started the day full of optimism but not everybody appeared to help me maintain a positive point of view.

I do have the mental agility to be good at putting shapes together because of it a talent lies within me to be good at dry stone-walling. Duke was astonished with the stone- wall I repaired. I expressed my creative talents to him. My energy level took a slight nose-dive everything seemed boring but I managed to show that I enjoyed doing it because I need praise and encouragement.

On February 16th Abbey gave birth to a baby boy, she named Theo. I went to visit them on Saturday with my mum at Hilltop Maternity Hospital. He was a small skinny baby he has dark brown hair and brown eyes. He will find an outlet for all the love I have for him inside of me. Jasmine is pregnant her baby is due in October.

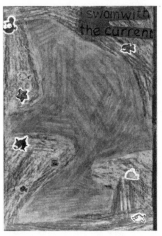

Whenever we did a cobble edge because we did a concrete path it was always my job to backfill with soil. Ada always laid most of the cobbles. When she stood over watching me work, I hated it. Duke seemed to be off hand with me every day because he did not let me do a lot of practical work. I found it hard to get on with them. I did everybody a favor by going out of my way to keep the peace. If I were assertive and made a fuss bad feeling would have lingered for at least a week.

We started work at a primary school on the housing estate. We did a cobbled edge for a tree seat duke and the other lads made. I got on with making a mulch path on my own. It gave my confidence a boost having a job to do. Other people got on with planting Rowan, Beech and Cherry shrubs.

A woman Health & Safety Officer came out to sight it was her job to access that we all wear protective clothing and is safety conscious so accidents will not happen. On that day, everybody took turns using the grass cutter. The people who were not operating it helped me wheelbarrow the sods to the corner of the field, dumped the grass there.

When it was just I, Duke, Ada, Fabian who was *a* volunteer on Haydn's team? Duke told me there is not enough work for me to rake the stone for the concrete path. He told me to sit and watch if I want. I felt offended when he treated me like an outcast. I took the spade off Fabian **so** I could rake the stone he helped *Duke* and Ada to load the stone from the tipper into a wheelbarrow they rotated wheeling the stone over to be tipped into the trench. I have a good eye for leveling. I did not do a good job of it to impress Duke or prove myself to him. He complimented me I am spot on it hurt because he did not appreciate me.

I liked it better when I worked on my own initiative because I did not have people watching over me or taking over. I resented Ada working with us because since day one Duke would never expect too much of me. I knuckled down under his orders, but still felt like he gained the upper hand. Jed a new lad started on the course another one who did not talk much. I felt very isolated because there was not anybody with a personality I could relate too.

I did not let the blip in proceedings impair my vision of an idea that was tailor-made for me. The picture shifted dramatically. I made fresh starts and resolutions not to let the grass grow under my feet. The time came to get more assertive and make changes. I encountered many challenges and met them with determination, battled through. Ada and Duke were obstacles placed in my path but I overcame them by using my own initiative. I did not wait to be asking what to do. It was more rewarding than I could ever imagine. I had a sense of duty and responsibility.

I got on with jobs on my own. I used a sander so I could sand graffiti off two benches. Stock fencing will replace the rotten fence everybody discarded off because it was falling to bits. I thought about the long run. I did not expect to finish the course get a job straight away. Ideally I would like to live in Hebden Bridge to be able to live there I need to find work in Calderdale. I hoped some peculiar happenings would turn to my advantage. What materializes will be a gift. The competitive side to my nature will definitely be stimulated. I will reach a higher level.

Melba arranged by phone to make an appointment with Magnus at the bank in Accrington. He worked there four times a week. On March 14, we went by taxi to see him. I finally had access to all of my money I did not want to tie anymore of it up into another account. He put my £3000 into my current account. Paper work with Magnus was now outdated. I brought a Sony television and Video. I brought a Sony music system. I needed to get renewal TV license. I joined the local gym. I gave my mum her £300 back she lent me for my storage unit. The bank sent me an application form for a credit card in the post, so I applied for one.

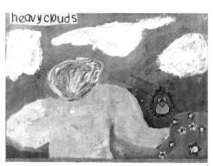

DARKENED LIGHT

I wanted to gear myself up to reach a higher level. Patsy and Gabby two students studying conservation did **their** work placement on Duke's team. Ada got a job working for the National Trust. I had a sore throat on Ada's last day. Duke dropped me off home. Over the weekend, Monday and Tuesday I could not eat because it made me sick. I spent most of my time in bed sleep was the best remedy to recover. On Wednesday, Mick and Vic took us all to Hoilingworth Lake in a mini bus. We had a look at the insects, wildlife the conservation side to it a walk around, the lake; some fresh air was just what I needed.

Over the next couple of days, I did not have any get up and go. I managed to dig a hole to put a post in for a sign Duke made. When everybody cleaned out the stream, planted aquatic plants I sat watched in the sunshine. I helped rake turf off a flowerbed to prepare for it to be block paved. Whenever Davy and Leo turned up for work there was a strange atmosphere because Duke pushed me to one side gave them my jobs to do. I decided to bide my time before I asked him what is wrong. Blake and Jed leveled mixed the cement. Leo and Davy leveled the sand and grit. When I had nothing to do, I got tension in my legs because I was not good at saying what I was feeling. The time came when I had to put myself, first. I was yawning faster than I could say I am bored.

SUSAN SPLAINE

On college day, I was not afraid to express my inner tensions to Duke or Margo. I got to grips with worries at work for the first time I showed hidden capabilities that is within my nature. Whenever Duke said I am spot on I ignored him I did not accept his praise because I was hurt. I did not let him hinder my progress. I was bursting to step out of myself. I had been waiting in the wings for a while, that made life rather slow going. I was not pushing myself forward. If I take the right steps to impress in the right, way I will not go far wrong. The green light shining that meant go. If I stretch my wings, I have the potential to show great forbearance.

Jude did nine weeks last summer: On April 25, he came back onto the team. He is an extrovert with a big personality. At last, somebody for me to connect with we got on. We started on a new site on the housing estate. It was waste ground that had not been managed, the grass on the footpath overgrown, a lot of litter accumulated. I was quite happy litter picking because I was not motivated to do hard graft. Blake and Jed litter picked, judging by the glum look on their faces they were not happy about it. Leo, Jude and Duke scraped the turf off the footpath. The kids were off school being verbally abusive. I ignored them because they were hard to cope with.

Haydn's team in Oldham were digging over gardens, to lay flags when he needed a helping hand all three teams joined forces. I usually removed debris from the gardens or did some digging. In the afternoon, the team leaders and all the lads played football I watched bored. I had not had an appetite. I was sleeping but still felt tired and edgy. My mind felt distracted. I joined the local gym for the psychological benefits. I cannot get any slimmer than I already am because I have accepted I am suited to the weight I am. Exercise speeds up my metabolism, increase mental endurance and my energy level.

I stopped going out with the British Trust because there were too many people and not enough work. Gabriel one of the older employees at groundwork was doing up gardens in the poor side of Heywood: Put new fencing up, flagged and block paved the drives. Only one volunteer Nigel worked with him. Duke's team sometimes worked with him because there was a lot of work to do. Gabriel did the flagging on his own. My mane jobs to do were digging holes for fence posts. I leveled the stone for flagging and did block paving.

On May 22, three new lads started on the course working with Gabriel, Cary, Clark and Gene. **Gene did** not like it he got very lethargic so he left. Gabriel has a sense of humour so I was able to break new ground with him. I shined working with Gabriel because I came out of myself a bit more. Two teams working together made light work of a heavy load.

SUSAN SPLAINE

On May 30 Aidan a volunteer started work on Duke's team. We spent a full week at a primary school in Oldham. We dug over the grass so Les another employee could do a cobble path. I could not hammer nails to join the bench seat to the legs. I did not do any of the steppingstones with flags. Two schoolchildren aged nine who lived across the road from the school they helped me paint the fence a blue colour.

It is through creativity I like to express myself; I had not been doing anything that was creative. I saw myself stood at the starting post because I wanted to move on in life but had nowhere to go. Intuition is what counts to me I will know when the time is right to put in my maximum effort. It is a long running saga for my active mind getting to many ideas. I do not stay focused on the here and now. We started work on another project at the school on the housing estate. We made an amphitheatre out of stone, did a cobble edge and some little steps, the sods we put into the corner of the field will be like a seating area.

DARKENED LIGHT

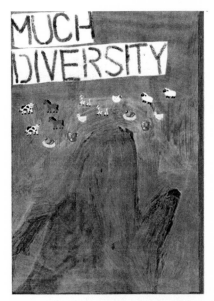

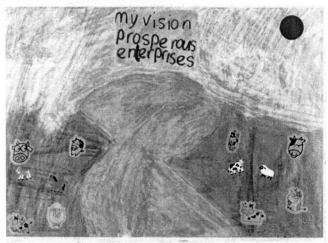

SUSAN SPLAINE

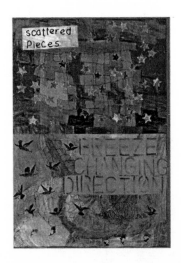

CHAPTER FOURTEEN

Over recent weeks, I had been enjoying work and getting along with people. Over night, I woke up and found it hard to make social contact with people. I felt withdrawn because I was within myself. I looked as if I am not interested in my work. In the morning I felt sick, butterflies in my stomach, I was inadequate. Siam is my New Deal Adviser because Sally has left. When she came to see me at the groundwork office for a review, I told her that everything is fine. For some reason of tact and diplomacy I kept my emotional health to myself, I took days off from the course because I could not be bothered to get out of bed in the morning. When I break with routine, I want to take flight. The distance traveled is of little importance the fact that I am on the move is all that matters. I want bigger and brighter days to lie ahead.

I think I felt depressive because memories of the last three months in Blackburn are at the forefront of my mind. I think I need to talk about Rojo she was the only person I did not get on with, me and Angus had our disagreements relationship became strained but it was not all bad. I had good relationships with every body else for us all to fall out just because I wrote a letter I think I needed to talk it through so I can find new ground because breakups are hard. I feel hurt because I was badly treated because I do not suffer from mental illness did not know how to deal with me when how I was behaving took a hold of my personality and took over my mind. Whenever I felt physically unwell, they just told me it was anxiety. Anxiety what about I do not think I am not a nervous person. I do not suffer from the feeling of dread and doom. I always felt agitated and angry whenever people told me you are stressed it is just anxiety. I wanted to lash out become destructive because they were wrong so wrong.

I went to the office at Shelter to pay my rent. Della asked me "how is work going." I told her I have not been today because I just woke up at four in the evening. Della understood where I was coming from and thought that I need counseling so that memories will fade from my mind. Melba arranged for me to see somebody at Victim Support to talk through traumas in my life. I needed to work on my pain I felt in my chest and in my throat. My head felt heavy because I found bad memories a strain I carried inside my head because I could not get rid of them.

The morning is the worst time of the day for me. I do not feel like eating or drinking coffee. I still do not need help to cope with life events that made me feel physically ill. I do not think trauma is having a long-term effect on me. I do not need psychotherapy so a therapist can delve into my subconscious. I think about who I am and I think about where I am at and going in life. Working my way through it will make me start to think more closely about my emotions and thoughts in general. I just want somebody to say it was wrong of them turning against me because I was not feeling very well talking to somebody about the last three months of my life at Seven Wonders. Melba went with me to Victim Support to arrange an appointment to see somebody. I listened to what Anne had to say. What I heard in a strange room was of great benefit. I expressed my feelings to them personal matters were now coming into focus. There have been occasions when the personal side to my life has been somewhat ignored. Time is on my side. I slowed down but I will get back on track.

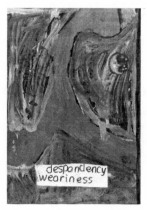

On Monday July 10, we worked in Heywood with Gabriel. I looked off colour because I was not motivated I did not have any energy. Duke gave me a lift home. I was lost in an emotional world of my own. It was the first time I saw my GP when Melba took me because she thought I should be on anti-depressants. She did not give me any medication I was glad about that because if she did I would not have taken them. She arranged for me to see a Community Mental Health Nurse. As I grow up change is apart of life and embrace in whatever I do.

Oona and Margo arranged for a Mentor to come and see me at groundwork. On Fridays after work, I saw Yvette at Victim Support now I see somebody else called Melba at groundwork office regularly. She is somebody I found easy to connect with, thinks I could reach my true potential if I keep my confidence and self-esteem at a high level. I had been skirting around for long enough. The time for action arrived. I wanted to fit in more than I was doing push forward progressively.

With a strimmer, Duke strimmed the long overgrown grass I raked up the grass with the other lads. Daisy from the Variety Going on Centre came to see me. She deals more with people who have come out of hospital, settling back into the community.

Gabriel went on holiday Duke was doing other things. His team worked with Les and Lain. I had to walk home from Rochdale because the buses were on strike. Walking down Drake Street I met Terry drinking cider on the wall outside the Hostel where he lived; a friend of his was also with him. He invited me to sit down talk to them. He gave me his mobile phone number. I let him walk me home invited him into my flat. Terry who was forty-five is the first ever white man to ever pick me up, because every body else were Asian well (apart from Ralph, Lorenzo and Robbie). He made a pass at me so I told him to leave he asked me if he did something wrong then he left me alone. I seem to attract deadbeats. Maybe it is because I am a deadbeat myself. An Asian man I met recently I gave him my address he came round to my flat and started masturbating. He told me that I am not a jackpot winner. His dad owns two restaurants he asked me if I wanted a job working in the bar. I could not work in a bar I am not very good at dealing with people. I do not understand what is it about me men keeping their brains in their pants. I do not have my brains in their pants and would not even want to touch them. I do not crave to be loved I can do without comfort and tenderness.

My moment will come when it is my turn to do well and I will, get what I want. A little patience and it will all work out for the best. It takes me a while to get myself fully into gear, but once I have done there really is no holding me back. Those things that take longer are all the better as a result.

The kids being off school was very easy for me to view it from gloomy prospective. Since Mick left, we had not been going to college every week. Working in Heywood I saddled myself with extra responsibilities, I pushed myself beyond the limits because I had the stamina. I still hated working on the housing estate in Oldham when we worked with Haydn. I did a lot of digging and got blisters on my hands. We also did fencing the job I hate the most because I cannot hammer nails. Jude got the sack because he took the week off did not phone Oona or Margo. I told Margo I am taking a couple days off because my back was sore.

Yvette at Victim Support was somebody I found easy to talk too. I was interested in how people grow up it is to do with their up bringing and environment. How people turn out to be, the way they are it is partly because of friends and people who had an influence over them. Self-discovery has been a solitary journey for me! I am far more capable than I think but in a working environment sometimes I want people to just ignore me, sometimes I join in using my own initiative.

How I Was as a child those personality traits are still a big part of me!

I live in a dream world.
I do not look at life realistically when I am making decisions and plans.
I succeed in imagination but not reality.
Slow thinker.
I tend to exaggerate or embroider the truth.
I am unduly when I am isolated, unsociable, withdrawn, solitary and distant. When I am in a happy mood, I am the complete opposite of isolation.
I lacking in self-confidence when I feel glum and miserable. When I am happy, I believe in myself and have confidence.
I am not easily taken advantage of I put myself in risky situations.
I get easily annoyed.
I am impulsive.
I want hope from suffering.
I want to be attracted to secure situations when searching for a new path.

Duke sacked Blake on July 1 because he took a lot of time off. I did not speak to Blake in the seven months I knew him. He did sometimes speak to me because he spoke in a quiet voice I did not respond. I absorbed his miserable mood. He made the day feel tense instead of lively. After his departure, I came out of myself more. I showed a different side to myself.

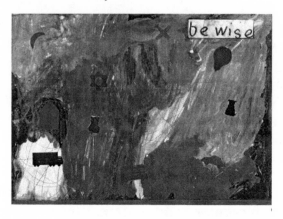

I wanted to immerse myself by doing something creative, express my talents. My mind ceased up because I was not getting any mental stimulation. We worked in big groups it made my mind distracted because I had nothing to do. Up above I could only see grey skies. On wet dreary days the day felt like it was not going to end. My sunlight darkened because I have not had enough horticultural experience to get a job. I need good luck stars to take me to wherever I will end up. A big boss needs to believe in me, give me a chance. He will be up there at the highest point of the summit when I reach the pinnacle. However, this depends on my part and on my ability to ride the waves of possibility when I come to the bottom of the mountain landscape that will eventually present it self.

DARKENED LIGHT

I cut up my credit card because I have gotten myself into debt again. The lightening broke my video I do not usually leave it plugged in, on that night I did. It had to be serviced cost me £50, my mum paid for it because I had to pay by a cashiers bankcard which I do not have. I did not pay her back.

On Tuesday August 29, Jude came back onto the course. It was another boring day when too many people worked together at a school in Whitworth block paving. Cast me to one side made me feel insecure and lacking in overall confidence in my skills as a landscaper.

When we did a concrete path on site on the housing estate in Rochdale, I made sure I had something to do. I took stock of my current progress, decided when it was time to have a rest. I increased the level of my skills because I could address a job that was tailor-made for me because I am good at path work. Relationships with people I worked with improved in leaps and bounds.

Karin a Mental Health Support Worker came *to* see me every Friday. She is a very over-powering, Amazon sort of woman she criticized because I am imperfect and have many faults. I went to my doctor's surgery because I had an appointment to see a Mental Health Nurse. I told her since childhood I have been suffering from black feelings of despair; my physical health is not that good. She arranged for me to see a psychiatrist.

Karin wants to get me involved in leisure activities and social groups. I built up some kind of defense barrister because of her comments about how I think and how feel do not match up because of what I am saying and my body language. She expected instant changes overnight. I felt as if she put me down I am the way I am because it is who I am. Personality traits I have might not be my true self but the real me will come out naturally in time. People like support workers seem to think that I am super human. I did not talk to her because she is not the right person who will take me in the direction where I want to go. Mixing with people who have mental health problems is not for me because I do not have mental health problems. My only problem is bad genetics. If my mum were not the way she was, I would be a normal whole person without missing links. I was not very open with her because she got snappy with me so I disappeared into a black hole that made her more annoyed with me. Maybe I did it to piss her off because she always seemed to be annoyed with me. I found her difficult to get along with so my difficult awkward side took over my personality most of the time when she came to see me.

Jude got a Job working for North West Water it was just me left with Duke because Jed finished his six months. I sometimes worked with Gabriel and With Haydn where

I hated it the most. Duke did not work with us all the time because he got a new job in the office I think as a designer. A site that needs doing up he plans it all out and decides what to do to improve the environment. I started a period when I began to feel at peace within myself.

Confidence should grow with time when things go my way. I have the potential to show a positive face to the world. I wanted to begin a journey in a completely new direction I had belief that I will cover new ground and learn many new things especially about myself and also discover hidden capabilities about what I am and who I am.

Haydn had been redundant because there was not enough funding left to finish of the work putting flags down in people's gardens. Duke finished of the work on the housing estate in Rochdale. It is only Gabriel left with a team so I worked with him, Cary and Clark; Nigel was not there anymore because he got a job I think working in a sports store. Gabriel took me under his wing until I came to the end of my course my last day October 13t. He kept me busy I doing my favorite job leveling stone for flagging.

On my last day Oona picked me up from Heywood, drove me to the office to see Melba my Mentor. Margo had also been redundant because groundwork is no longer doing training courses. If I want to live in Hebden Bridge, she advised me to write to the Council in Calderdale asking for employment and accommodation. Melba also advised me to go to the job centre in Halifax. When Gabriel unloaded the tools at the office in the basement, he gave me a lift into Rochdale Town Centre with Cary who wants to carry on working with Gabriel as an employee until he has finished all of the gardens. The only way that matters now is forward! I did not celebrate finishing the end of course. I felt tired so tired I had an early night. In October, Jasmine gave birth to a baby boy Topsy he looks just like Sid.

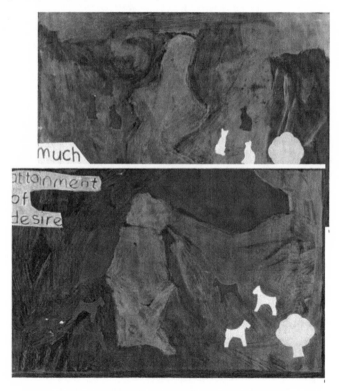

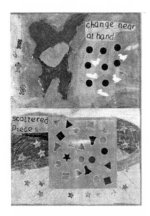

CHAPTER FIFTEEN

Personal projects came to a grinding halt. I expected it would be hard to get things moving again. I had to be realistic try not to escape into a fantasy world. I had far fetched dreams moving to Hebden Bridge. I want the ambience to be beautiful green scenery, a village and a canal. I put effort into finding work by going to the job centre in Halifax, and going to the housing office. I asked the receptionist if she would give me the address of personnel department at the council, so I could write letters if they have any jobs. Every two weeks they sent me job bulletins through the post but never did have any horticultural jobs. I left some space for myself to think over the past two years. I have gained the impetus and skills that will make me a good candidate to get employment. My financial state was depressing because I do not have much money to spend on treats on myself.

I went to the job centre to sign back on the dole for three months Sian my New Deal Adviser helped me with job search. She wrote to garden nurseries and Garden Center's in Calderdale. An employer for a garden company in Todmorden wrote me a letter stating that I should write back to him in March because there is not much work in winner and autumn. Spring and summer is the season for gardening.

I put a lot of thought into what I want from life. Achieving and progress was my number one priority. When Sian did attempt to push me into work I did not want to do I was not willing to listen to help that was proffered because it was not in the direction where I wanted to go. It might be in March when job opportunities will give me an added incentive to play to win because I do not like being a loser. I come from a family of losers I want to be above them so I can look down on them.

When Karin came to see me she was always voluble said what she thought about my slow

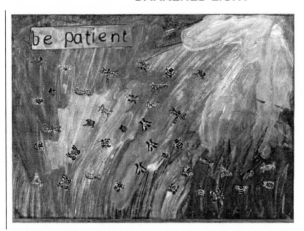

progress into finding work and about my social skills because I have low self-esteem. I did not care about social skills. What she wanted me to do was to talk non-stop about my boring week and bore her to tears because I have not done anything exciting. All that mattered to her I should get out and mix with people who have psychiatric problems. I lived with people with psychiatric for three years, now I want normal people in my life because I get on and click with people who are not mental. I did not bother telling her because she would have disagreed with me and had one of her heated debates with herself. It is usually men in a position of authority I click with and can relate too because I do click and make a connection with men and not women.

Karin tells me that I think about the past. I do not live in the past because I am a cold person and can live my life as if the past does not hurt. I am not in denial, emotionally and mentally I am not affected by everything that as gone on. People suffer from reactive depression and nervous illness because they live in the past. I do not think I ever suffered from anxiety. I do not suffer from the feeling of dread and doom. My body does not shake my lips do not tremble because I do not get into nervous states. I am in denial I get depressed because over the year's professional people like therapist/support workers have told me it is just stress and anxiety. I have never told anybody I feel depressed. What happened in November ninety-four I do not see it as a bad experience. I do need to look back and talk about my past because I do not suffer from reactive depression because I do not pity myself. I need to talk about why I suffer from psychosomatic symptoms: I want doctors, nurses, mental health workers to stop telling me it is stress and anxiety because it annoys me; they are wrong, so wrong.

I have not let my past hinder my future feeling, as if I do not want to live because trauma happened to me: Pitiful people only go out to go shopping and to day centers, stay in all day thinking about the bad times that is why they get depressed. They do not want to live and do not have any ambition in life. Rewards have come to me because of my past efforts. The progress I made depended on timing. Whatever was on my mind unfolded in good time because I did not give up I have patience because I have good insight.

I do not want to get out of bed in the morning

when my mind is full of fog because time goes by dead slow.   When I do not eat enough I am sluggish because my metabolism slows down.   I went to the gym in the evening but I did not feel revitalized after it because my energy level was low. I spent *days* **walking and** going **into town not to buy nothing because I did not have any money.**

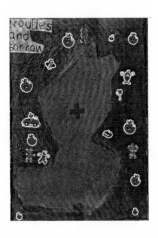

I told Karin that I am reluctant to go to my **mum's house for** Christmas. When I attend family gatherings, I feel like an outsider because I do not fit in or belong I told Karin ideally I would like to go to a hotel. She responded by saying if I do I need to talk to people there talking is all that mattered to her and it annoyed me. Why should I initiate conversation when all I want is some peace and be by myself. I am out of a job so people would have looked down at me if I did go because I had the money. I like to have time on my own and my Quiet moments but it does not mean I like being lonely and my own company. When I reached the age of fourteen, I did not a get presents every year. When I went back to school, pupils talked about what they got, said to what I got for Christmas I replied nothing. I remember Abbey looking at me laughing because she wanted me to say I got this and that just like she did. She was the liar and I was the truthful one. .

I hated life so much I wished I had never been born. My mum and dad should not have had kids because they could not give encouragement or praise so we will make a future and a better life *for* ourselves. They were unhappy with their own lives. Ernie was not disappointed in Jasmine because she is trashy and a bit of a tramp just like him.   Zandra does not see Paddy as a big disappointment because he does not want to work and is spending all of her money. What will he live of when it has all gone? Zandra will still get her pension every month. When Theo goes to school will Abbey try get back into work because what will she do all day. I do get tired of stop- gaps, feeling restless waiting for something new and interesting to happen. I have a humdrum existence but I believe it will not be like this forever once I reach my mountain landscape. When I climb to the top to paradise, my life will be a beach and a bed of roses.

It is hard to feel happy when for far too long I

have been woebegone. I need to be hearty about something I can hold onto and believe in besides writing my book. I need a passion in life that will take me to earthly paradise, surrounded by orange scenery. I hoped and wished that life will offer me new incentives and the chance to do whatever takes my fancy in other ways.

Karin regularly took me out to Tesco for a soft drink. We sat at the table had a chat. I tried to be optimistic so that she would not lecture me about being more positive. . She still criticized me because I was not open or forthcoming with her. She gave me a lift to my mum's house because I needed £10 to get some food she gave me the money when Paddy was not in the lounge. On Tuesday December 12, I could not go to the cinema with Karin and her son, somebody she worked with because I only had enough money for necessities. She understood I was a recluse on the dole. I was feeling as if that black cloud is above my head. Any departure from my boring routine would fill me with excitement. I went to the gym on a cold rainy night because I had a weekly bus ticket.

On the bus coming home, the dark haired and dark eyed bus driver set my heart a-flutter, because I do find dark people attractive. I think the bus driver just started a new job because he was not wearing his uniform. He was wearing a bright red shirt, and black Jeans. It was pouring down with rain so heavy when I got off the bus he said he could not see out the window. I did not look at him or say anything. Whenever I went to the gym, he always seemed to be the bus driver. I think he worked shifts at two different times because whenever I walked down Manchester Road either going to town or walking back home, I used to see him driving past me.

Karin repeatedly kept on telling me I am not aware of my body language. I did not care about my posture because I did not have a job and my days are empty. I felt so lost within myself. She tells me I look vulnerable as if I am from another planet. I was not always aware when I was being unresponsive. She felt uncomfortable because I would not make eye contact with her. I did not invite her in when she came to see me that was because I do not have manners. I reached the point I did not want her to come and see me anymore so I did not make a connection. She treated me as if I am a waste of space so I do not know why she bothered coming.

Over recent weeks, I had been getting headaches regularly. I do not know why I was crying when she came I had to say something so I told about dreams I was having, being in a dark tunnel, four shadowy grey figures hovering above me I think it symbolized Hope, Rojo, Tukishi and Jeremiah. I found it hard to dismiss images from the forefront of my mind. I felt barricaded within myself because of concealed feelings. I stayed in bed until the afternoon. I have left Seven Wonders with a fear of confrontations and showdowns, because memories will come into my mind of the showdown I had with four bitter people. I do my best to keep the peace and not make people angry with me. I do sometimes lose control of myself and become reckless and impulsive because of my behaviour people get annoyed with me so they will confront me. I don not want to remember times that hurt. I do not feel hurt but maybe I do need to talk about why was everybody so angry with me because I do not understand. I will not be able to learn or change behaviour that makes people so angry with me because I do not know what made them tick.

Karin phoned up my GP because she thought I should be taking anti-depressants I did not say to her I feel depressed but she took over. Karin went with me to see the GP, as if I imagined she would not give me anti-depressants because I am not a depressive. Karin made the wrong decision for me to go to the doctors so she took her frustration out on me. Repeating her, I just need help with social skills and with my confidence, self-esteem. What she saw on the outside I do not see on the inside. I see a character that is crafty, scheming. Shrewd and cold stone because she does not show remorse, feel guilt and does not have a conscience. If a criminal mastermind taught her how to be a con artist, I think she will be good at it and would not go to prison because being crafty comes natural to her.

I let her read the chapter when I finally ran off from Seven Wonders. Next time when she came to see me, she thought that I gave Hope and her merry men so much power. Hope and Rojo would not let go of their anger there was not nothing I could do to avoid their bitterness. I had an image inside my head when I get my money out off the interest account then I will be out of there. She did not explain to me why I gave them so much power and control over me. Karin compared my book to a Catherine Cookson novel because there is a lot of despair in it.

She was very critical that I repeated some thoughts that are because it was not finished and I did not have the patience typing it all out. I had thoughts inside my head that I will borrow a computer of somebody and rewrite my chapters in a different format leaving out my repeated thoughts, and how I sometimes describe myself that is not the real me because I listen to my inner voice. She also said thoughts I have written does not sound like me. I sometimes feel as if it is not me thinking but my inner self-taking over my mind. I did not stand my ground when she was being ruthless because she thinks I am naïve. There is not any right or wrong in what people think about how I write, this book is not a diary I have wrote it being reflective and writing down my thoughts. Her comments did not hurt me because she can be dim I saw it as one of her faults because she does not look beyond comprehension. She did not always understand where I was coming from and I could not always understand where she was coming from. Whenever Karin could not see, my point of view she would create a tense situation because she had heated debates with herself. When I could not see her point of view, I just ignored her.

I mentioned to her that Sidney was critical of me because I do not have a boyfriend. I do not think having a boyfriend would make my world a much better place. My book is about my life it is also my life until I have finished it. At this point in my life, I am not even thinking about relationships because I do not have anything to show for myself. I think he should be critical of him self, being in a relationship with somebody who does not like him. Jasmine and Sidney are both rough so their kids will be rough. I could not understand why he was having a go at me, in comparison to Abbey I do not want to be on my own with a child. I think Sidney should have been critical of her because she does not take Theo out anywhere to places kids like to go, his childhood is not about having fun and innocence. If I were a single mum, I would not stay in every Sunday and only take the child out grocery shopping. . Sidney had no right criticizing me because I do not have kids I cannot afford to look after. He criticized me insinuating that I am a lesbian. Karin would not listen to me because she was very firm in her opinions; I just ignored her because I am ignorant All Karin had to say was she is on her own with a child and so are many other women. What I was trying to say to her is Sidney thinks I should have a relationship with somebody who I cannot stand the sight of, be lumbered with a kid, because I split up from the father because I felt miserable with him. Nevertheless, it is not what I want. I will not have any because I might pass on bad genetics. I do not want to bring a child into the world because it might suffer the same way I did and just stay mute.

In March, I felt optimistic because I thought I might get a job. I wrote back to the Garden Company in Todmorden.   I applied for a job at the Garden Centre near by. On the job front, nobody replied to me. I had the drive to apply myself to recover lost ground. I wanted to make contacts in what is to me a brave new world that will fill me with optimism. To feel self-satisfied I wanted a sense of responsibility, industry and determination to achieve. In a workplace, I have proved to myself to be capable of carrying a heavy load at work. My life was not speeding up for a reason. I was keen to chase a few potential rainbows.   That crock of gold was elusive I was beginning to think is it there at all.

The best thing for me to do is just keep on traveling and be grateful for the points I do win. Making a **niche** for me with my book when it is finished me will be doing something worthwhile during the day. My progress obstructed because I have not come to my mountain landscape just yet, so I waited in the wings for my time to come. I concentrated on endeavors that will had to my own happiness. That mountaintop is miles out of sight. In the far distance inside my head, I can still see that light of hope flickering.

My GP made an appointment for me to see a psychiatrist. Karin came with me so she could take over about what she thinks my needs are. All he was interested in was my childhood. He thinks I should go to Mental Health Centers and do gardening. I wanted to talk to him because I am uncertain what my true nature is. I do not know how to describe myself. There are issues I need to discuss why I still put myself in situations where men might hurt me. I do not know why I behave the way I did. In November 1994 I let two men hurt me because I schemed, plotted, hatched a ploy to get out of the house. Imperfection brought me sickness and sorrow because hatred drove me. I craved what is bad. I want to do what is right now so I will not cause people pain. My conditions on earth were not conflict that went on within me. I wanted good things for myself. I taught myself to create harm and pain for myself, so I could change my life because I did not know any better. I chose to be treated badly it was worth the pain because I thought it was the course of action that would bring me lasting happiness. There are things I want to talk about in confidence. The secret I am carrying around inside me it is not a burden but I feel as if I need to tell somebody.

My mum gave me £20 a month to pay for my television license. Karin made an appointment for me to see a Benefit Adviser at a Mental Health Centre about claiming incapacity benefit. Then Karin told me I would not get a sick note because I just need help to be assertive and improve on my social skills, myself-confidence, and self-esteem needs building up because it is low. She wanted to help me with behaviour management. How I live, my life does not matter to nobody else. I have my needs: Food, shelter and warmth. If I reach my true potential, it would mean for me a miserable future or a happy one. Nobody wants to suffer or have troubles. I have made decisions about changing my life. What I wanted to do was broaden my horizons and carry on working towards finding work. I do get through things I see as being important. There will be peace in my world when a new path of fulfillment opens. I want my world to be a much more glamorous place to live in.

I ask myself what difference does staying good make if you want to be bad. The time came for me to leave Shelter Melba had been off sick, so Doris applied for housing with St.Vincent's. Living in a flat on my own will not **suit me** down to the ground. On my own, I will not be able to put all of my resources into making all of the right moves when the timing is right to take me into a different direction. I wonder about the huge sky filled with stars at night. I admire the beauty of the countryside. There must be a grand purpose in al

DARKENED LIGHT

these things. Where am I going? Is there more I can expect? Feeling dissatisfied with life reflects how frayed I feel around the edges. Life is not paradise on earth. I want a measure of life and happiness before I die. I am wishing upon a star.

Amber, an Occupational Therapist from the Variety Going on Centre came to my flat, to give me information about outdoor activity group at the Rochdale Lake in May. Karin arranged for me to take part in it with people who suffer from mental disorders. I was prepared to show a flexible face when I do the six week outdoor pursuit course. I was sure of me I am capable doing the activities. I did not want to fail because I needed praise. I do not see Karin anymore because she has moved on to pastures new. I was glad about that because she did nothing but insult me in my face. On the course, I will be doing team building exercises, canoeing, and kayaking, sailing, indoor climbing. I missed map reading because I went to Blackpool with Abbey and Theo.

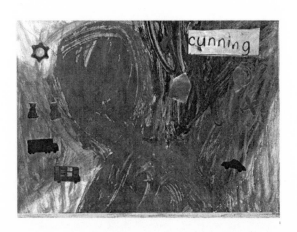

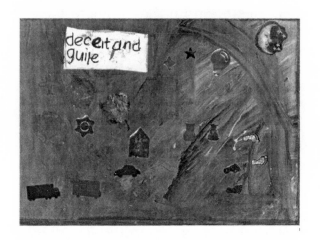

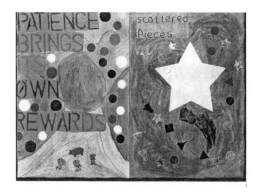

CHAPTER SIXTEEN

During the summer in June two thousand and one, I went out for a wonder. At about six thirty in the evening I used to see the same bus driver pass me buy. Bus spotting watching him pass by became one of my favorite pastimes. It was my instincts telling me when he would pass me by, feeling the need to leave the house and walk down the road. I did not stick to a particular course of action walking the streets just so he would crop up every time I left the house. It was not just in the evening but also afternoons. I love to be around men who are funny, interesting and stimulating. Asian men seem to like me, but I do not want relationships with Asian men. I tend to be much talkative than is expected of me because men with a sense of humour lighten the load somewhat. There was a sense excitement and optimism being generated but I was not sure why. I believe listening to my intuition plays an important part in life because it can lead you in the right direction. If something is destined to happen then it, will.

Melba came back to work after being off sick for four months. She felt it was her duty to help me find voluntary work. I was at the starting post and I needed help from unexpected quarters. It was hard for me to get anything done in a concrete sense on my own. I wanted to retain my self-esteem. I cannot forge ahead create the kind of life I want by myself. I got splinters in my feet because my trainers had slits in their souls. Walking boots were uncomfortable to wear all day. I fell over with my shoes on in town. My mum brought me a new pair of adidas trainers. I was financially dependent on her to give me money for food when my cupboards, freezer and fridge were empty. Paddy erupted like a volcano but I did not care about his feelings. He was not miserable married to Ernie for years and years. It is not even his money so he should not be spending it. Melba applied for Disability Living Allowance because since 94 I have felt physically ill. I have problems with my sleeping and motivation. I do get tired living an empty life and being retreated from the outside world.

DARKENED LIGHT

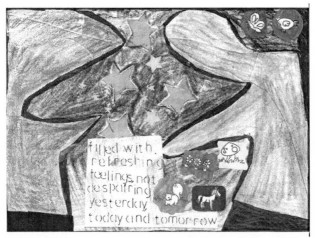

filled with
refreshing
feelings not
despairing
yesterday
today and tomorrow

I hung onto the hope, standing beneath my light of hope that opportunities lied ahead for me. Each day is a step closer to where you want to go. I hoped I will get the support I need to move onto a much more comfortable level of life when I come to the end of this road reach the finishing line, then get onto a new open road. My tenacity keeps me hanging on. I am right to feel there is more I can achieve. Anything that requires creative output will go exceptionally well. I am aware of my finer qualities and know how to project myself. When my objectives and aims are on target, I am very impetuous. Melba phoned up the Garden Centre who sent an application form because there were vacancies. By the time I filled in the application form, took it to the store the job had already gone. I needed a Guardian angel to fall down from the sky, reach for a star on my behalf that will take me down the road to a much more contented life. I will not mind fairies at the bottom of the garden waving magic wands.

St. Vincent's Housing offered me a flat on an estate near where Jasmine lives.   An Asian Housing Officer showed Melba and me around the one bedroom flat.   The flat had new kitchen units fitted in.   I will get an allowance to paint the kitchen wall. I signed my tenancy to move in on September 3. I felt jittery because I needed money for carpets, bedroom furniture, sofa, fridge and cooker.   I had an image inside my mind of myself living in squalor. It is destination where I will fit in and belong.   I did not say anything about my doubts and uncertainty.   I had this vision of my life staying in staring at the same four walls. My choices should count when I have a sense of direction.   Whenever I went to my mum's house because I did not have any food it was like a battlefield.   She kept on asking me do I have the social sent you a grant yet.   She expected me to move into an empty flat.   Sleep in my sleeping bag and sit on the cold floor.   She got overwrought about my impending mood. She worries about inconsequential matters.   I just ignored her.   The strain began to show because I shut down.   I could not do anything too remedy the situation.   All that mattered to her is I will not have to walk it from where I lived to her house anymore.   I did not complain because walking was the only exercise I did.

Darcy who worked at Shelter helped me transport some of my belongings in her car. Driving down the road, I saw that bus driver. We also went into two carpet stores. The staff at Shelter thought that I was able to live off £50 a week and have enough left over for cheap food. They are far from wrong and were being unrealistic. I received £260 from the social fund. Darcy appealed in writing a letter because I am hard done by. The staff at Shelter shared thoughts and ideas with each other about me; they thought I would not succeed on my own. It was the decision I made to stay there a little bit longer until I move into alternative accommodation. It would have been foolish of me to ignore new openings and opportunities. I could not afford to be vague or airy-fairy. I wanted my direction in life and outlook to change so I can find some comfort. As a period of change loomed I wondered whether or not if I would cope. I still needed to make discoveries about myself.

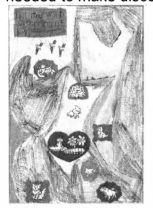

When I move forward positively I will fill in gaps in my life I plodded along until I am on the verge of a new beginning. I hoped somebody up there does like me; enrich my life. I waited for changes to happen when I move on in life. I desired a change in my fortunes because I do not want to live an incomplete life. I needed to find a new unseen benefit, make great headway then head for the hills. I want something to come from the rainbows I have been chasing. I had to carve out a place for myself anything to be successful has to be lasting.

The first scattered pieces of my life I drew I put it in chapter five. I drew one for each chapter because I want George to write a song titled scattered pieces. George is the light shining on my journey through life, because in ninety. Ninety-six his mellow songs inspired me to see life as a fortune journey on my earthly adventures. I want him to write the song as a theme tune to my book. It will be of significance, meaning and his purpose to have a big selling song that is heart-rending. We both will gain and triumph because of creativity and imagination despite our heaviness and cares. He is my golden influence to go for silver and gold. It will give us both added incentive to play to win. He is not dynamic anymore but he is in a position to force circumstances to work in my favor by helping me move my long-range plans a step closer to fulfillment.

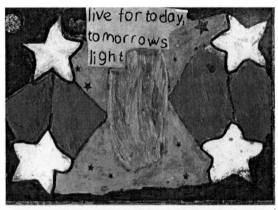

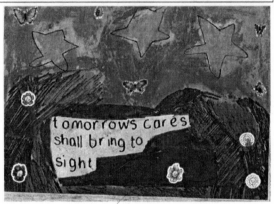

I came to the realization that I have access to something desirable. My obsession with him as put me in a mischievous frame of mind. I want us to be of great use to each other. I will do what I can to get close to him. I need his generosity, and he needs my special sort of kindness. This is a chance of a lifetime. It is possible however; he will have me in his sights as a potential candidate for something desirable and wonderful. My practical ideas will win him universal approval. He will put his creative talents to some use because it will sure to workout. The release of the song and the publication of my book we will be a truly unstoppable combination. He will hover in my spotlight because he will not overshadow me.

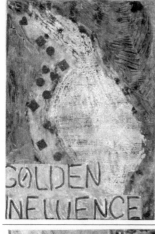

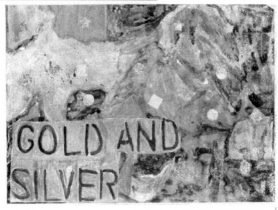

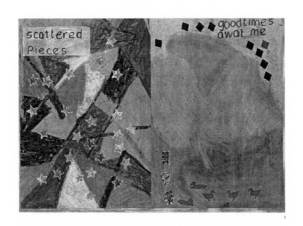

CHAPTER SEVENTEEN

On October 5, I attended a therapy group at a day centre for people with Mental Health issues. The group started at 12.00am and finished at 1.00pm; every Friday for twelve weeks. The group was into its third week when I started going. The group leaders were Ida who is the Manager of the Centre. Sari was a social worker student. Tony was the youngest person there. The four people other there Sonia, Vida, Art and Egan were in their late forties to mid fifties. Most of the people had mental disorders because of trauma, and bad experiences. Egan, Vida and Sonia do not get out much. I felt as if a bolt of lightning struck me because they were not my cup off tea. I felt out of place.

Egan complained about staying home too much because he is dissatisfied with life. He does not have the impetus to do something about it. I did not talk much in the group because I could only relate to Sonia; she talked a lot about her tormented childhood. Sonia also talked about daughter's suicide because her soldier boyfriend died in the gulf war. We all sat in a circle on chairs. I found it daunting because there was not anywhere to look but down. Whenever I made eye contact with somebody, I laughed. If everybody had the same life experiences that brought him or her to have therapy, I think I would have given more input. Art who is originally from Mauritius I could see from the corner of my eye, that he looked in my direction often. He smiled at me that made me feel uncomfortable, because I did not return his overtures.

I had seen Art previously in the waiting room when I went for a referral interview. He wanted a sympathetic ear because he had a headache. I was too engrossed inside my own head so I did not show him much concern. When the group finished after my first session he gave me a flash of his charming smile as I was leaving, he asked me out on a date. I turned him down because I did not have an appetite. I felt like I was looking inward, instead of outward. I needed to wake up from my reverie about me not being I, but somebody else because I hate myself because of one failing I have. Art is not the perfect man I would like to make a love connection with because we are not compatible. There is not a spark between us that will blossom into burning passion. Chemistry makes two people happy together. I am taller than he is. I do not think I hurt his pride because I was not interested in him. On Thursday afternoon before going to the next group I sat in a pub; hoping he would ask me out again. He will be just a whim because I am bored of being a recluse. I did not fancy him or find him attractive. I had mental images that tomorrow night I might be in a pub with him...

Art sat next to me in the group. Whenever I said something, he was the first to respond to me. He made comments how nice I looked when I smiled. When the group finished he asked me out on a date. I said I would go so he gave me a lift home. He was at University doing a nursing training course. He said he would pick me up at 7.30pm. I felt unruffled about my date. He did not brighten up my life. I told Tilly; she felt excited for me. He did not smite me. It was not love, never mind love at first sight. You need to fall for a person to fall in love.

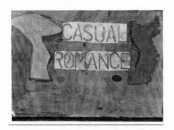

At about 6.30pm I had a bath, put on going out clothes I have had for other a year. Della styled my hair and put make-up on me. She even took a photograph. Art complimented on how nice I looked. He drove me to his cottage because he wanted to change his shirt. He lives in a shit hole his house is in need of repair. In the lounge, he has one leather chair. There were a lot of books and clutter on display. He should have a clear out but he will not get rid of anything. The cooker and microwave covered in grime and grease. He does not cook in the kitchen because he has his meals at University and eats out every night. The cupboards and draws were falling of their hinges. He is not independent-minded because he does not take care of himself. He cannot do household chores. His ex-girlfriend did his laundry. He is such a revolting man living in an unhygienic house. His only attraction was his black Honda jeep. He worked has a children's Health Visitor; every month he gets a pension from his old workplace.

He took me for a curry where he went regular on his own. He proudly showed me off to the waiter, the manager of the restaurant came out to talk to him. I had drunk martini and lemonade. Later on in the evening, we went to Chicago Rock Café club. I am not a party person so I felt bored all night. I never seem to do whatever it is I want to do. So I think I would much rather stay in bored. I am a theatre person and want to go out to comedy and jazz clubs. I managed to project myself and shine. I gave him the impression everything was going satisfactory because I were lively. I felt as if the wind of change filled me with fresh enthusiasm. He invited himself back to my flat for a cup of coffee. My stuff packed in boxes in the lounge. I dismantled my shelf unit he asked what it is so I told him shelves. He said he would like to see me again but did not set a date. During the week, he turned up on my doorstep.

I had a belief that I am frigid because I have never experienced sex in a loving way. What Ronald did to me is my earliest childhood memory. During my childhood, other people have stimulated sex with me. I remember two sisters Tessa and Dawn they had a friend called Yvonne. In the evening when my mum was out at Marge's house these three girls in their late teens came round to the house. My dad let them in just so they could show me their vaginas. I was just a child at primary school. I have a vivid memory of being on my bed with Dawn she pulled her knickers down, stroked herself. She got hold of my hand and made me touch her. I also have a vivid memory of Tessa stood up on her feet in the lounge in front of the closed door; she lifted up her skirt and pulled her knickers down; Yvonne sat me down on the floor underneath Dawn legs she kneeled down behind me, kept on pushing my head towards Tessa's vagina. Ernie sat in his easy chair watches them abuse me. I also remember somebody else I knew called Thea who was also in her late teens.

She took her clothes off in front of me in my bedroom. My mum came in shouted, told her to leave the house. She has a brother Tex who is a few years older than I am. I remember going into a block of flats, I with him standing in front of the disposable shoot he pulled his pants down told me to stroke him and gave him a blowjob. I also remember inside a ditch on a local field a local boy stimulated sex with me. We both kept our clothes on but he did lye down on top of me.

The repressive fear I have about sexual intercourse comes from bad experiences. Art brought alcohol to drink in my flat just so he could try to get me into bed. He made a pass at me. I did not give myself to him as a whole person. I would not let him penetrate me. I did not want to see his bare body never mind touch me. I did not keep my brains inside his pants. He told me he would like to see me again as he was leaving. His offers of social gatherings appealed to me quite naturally. I was not misery behind happiness being with him because I need something for I that is worthwhile and makes me feel self-satisfied. I had self-belief that I will emerge with self-confidence that withered away and build on it. I could see ahead to that time for me when I am not dark or lonely. I had a discussion with Art about my sexual experiences as a child left me scarred. He wanted to counsel me about it; tried to enlighten my doubts that left me unsure for all these years.

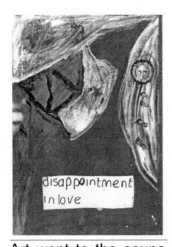

Art went to the sauna after university every day. He came round to my flat between 9.00pm-10.00pm every night. My time revolved around me staying in waiting for him to come. He left by 11.00pm because there is a rule visitors have to leave by 11.30pm. I did not look forward to seeing him. I did not think about him all the time. I did not want to be with him all the time. He wanted to be about togetherness all we have are each other. He was very touchy, liked cuddles and giving me finger jobs. I was not warm or loving in responses because I did not love him. I did not feel the need to give him physical affectionate, because passion and chemistry was not there between us. I did not give him cuddles but he gave me snuggles. He was not the worth of my life. I took care not to promise the earth because at that stage, I did not have good faith if I could come up with the goods. It is liberating to feel so positive, but I tried not to get ahead of myself because my active mind goes into overdrive. Gains are possible if I will just be patient.

On Mondays, I went to another group at the day centre. Jane who ran the group was a year younger than me. Several times, it was just her and me. We had conservations, which were just casual as if we were in a pub. I was full of warm feelings towards her because I found the atmosphere relaxing. I talked a lot about my journey of self-discovery. I felt frustrated trying to find work but to no avail. I learnt it is not how far you fall that counts but how high you bounce back. Practically every word spoke listened to closely. The fog lifted because minor changes took place in my life because of it I began to see blue skies. I had plenty of vision, new ideas and plans I wanted to put into action.

In October, Melba took me to the local nature reserve for an interview to begin voluntary work. Only two young men worked there. A woman is the secretary. A man worked there who liked watching musicals. He had an evening out in Manchester, watched Jesus Christ Super Star. I need a friend in my life who likes watching musicals so we could have nights out at the theatre. I only did tree felling for two days because the job centre referred me to the local job club. Melba also took me to a housing project. It is like a big house with six single flats in it. One woman works there during the day. There were not any vacancies so Melba wrote to another housing project. I filled in referrals forms just in case a vacancy may come up. Leaping forwards sounded much better. There is not an office on site; but the people who run the project do home visits during the evening. I was in a far-sighted mood, willing to get on in life and store up goodwill. New relationships coming into my life seemed to be on the cards.

After the sixth week of the group, Art stopped going because he went to university for his dinner instead. He was puffed up with his own importance. He could not stop telling me how wonderful I am. My dearest wish is something money cannot buy: Happiness, love, warmth and security. Art was on about taking me to Mauritius in spring. He is one of eight children, one sister and six brothers. His dad died in the army at the age of 42. His mum and most of his family live in Mauritius he also has family in Paris. Conditions applied to my life that would not have suited me down to the ground. I wanted to build happiness up on my misfortune. The two of us were not compatible. I was sure of myself I would get out of this relationship healthier and stronger.

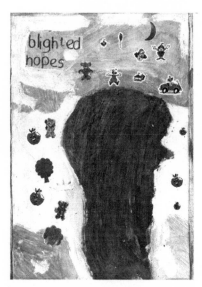

blighted hopes

I went in the afternoons to the job club because Jason worked in the afternoons. I was able to assert myself with him because I like men with dark brown hair and eyes. I decided to throw in the towel; stop going to the job club when I have done another Curriculum Vitiate and send letters to companies, enquiring about vacancies. If an employed replies to me I think people with influence will be impressed by my industry, application and will want to go out of their way to reward me for it. A job will have a positive effect on my income, and me even though I will only get the minimum wage.

I watched a programmed on television about actors who are heartthrobs. I am not sure why but a clip of a boy in the eighties, who was an antique expert on Terry Wogan's chat show; was on television he is now woman I had a conversation with Art because I do not like being a woman. If I was a man, I think I would be gay, because of my thinking I find myself attracted to gay men. I will not have a sex change. Art expected answers that did not seem right to me just yet. It would be wise to talk about it and seek some advice. As a woman, I am not deluded about my sexuality because I would not suck on a woman's breasts or lick out her vagina.

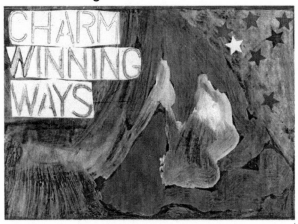

Art drove me to his house to show me some books about woman men. I wanted to watch sheltering the sky because John Malkovich was in it. Art got sexually excited and took me to bed. He did not arouse me. It hurt when he penetrated me because I was not moist. I did not feel at ease at all. I was never in the mood for romantic gestures with him. A full-blown love affair did not develop between Art and me. In a loveless relationship, you cannot promise each other the earth. In hell, hopes will shatter along with broken promises. My heart did not beat or flutter just for him. I was permissive because I did not want to be with him. I should have ended it. I could not bear to look at his face never mind his stomach.

He borrowed a laptop computer of a woman from university because she had five. I asked him if I could borrow it so I could type up my book; save it on disc. I strung him along because of my false feelings he thought were real. I think good luck will fall down from the sky into my lap where a publisher is concerned. I believe in what I want to achieve will happen. My positive aspect is success using my talents. It is hope I have held onto that keeps traveling. Melba received a reply back from Leaping Forwards. A man has moved out so there is a spare flat for me to move into as soon as possible. I waited for Melba to goad an appointment, then go and view the property. I saw myself at the stage in my life where I felt the need for change. I am in a galaxy where pigs can fly in never land of nod. It is just fantasy when I am in the midst of transcendental experiences. When a click wagon comes to town, I jump on it, and go on a white-knuckle ride.

Tudor and Ebony are the founders of leaping forwards. On Monday November 19 at 7.30pm, he picked Melba and me up at Shelter. He drove us to the flats that are located behind a curry restaurant-Hot &Spicy. The owner of the flats, offices underneath the flats and the restaurant is Mr. Caneek. The car park in front of the flats and at the back of the restaurant is Caneek Square named after him. The flat vacant for me to move into a dentist used to live there. The flats are within a community. Hugo and Almira were the only people apart of the project. People who did not have any mental problems or special needs occupied flat one, two and six. To get to the flats we have to walk up a flight of stairs. I was worried how we would get my television up there. We all went into Almira's flat who I already knew because she lived at Shelter. I found Ebony exhilarating because she is to get on with because she has a sense of humour. She does not take herself too seriously and does not behave as if she is a sergeant Major just because she is in a position of authority. Almira thinks the world of Ebony. I found Tudor staid because he came across to me as being thoughtful, calm and composed. I think he might understand I might not sometimes have control over my impulses when I have stupid moments. He will not react the same way everybody in Blackburn did and social workers by having showdowns and have heated debates why are people angry with me. Tudor is not domineering so he will not take over my life, make decisions for me because I can think for myself. People had no right telling me what to because what I wanted and what they wanted for me were both different things. When people take over and do not listen to me, relationships become strained.

The flats have two bedrooms. I want to use my spare room as a painting room. I also want to put the laptop computer Art borrowed in there because he wanted to help me type it up on computer but he does not think the same way as I do so if I let him tell me how to write it, it would not be my work. If I leave the computer in the lounge, he will sit next to me watching me type and take over. When I am upstairs on the computer, he will stay downstairs watching television so he will not watch over me and stress me out.

The housing scheme pays furnishing for the flats. I needed curtains, bedroom furniture, fridge and a suite and coffee table. Ebony and Tudor work during the day. I think Tudor is a mental health worker. Ebony as had a different variety of jobs. Tudor also gets itchy feet and moves from place to place. Monday to Friday from; 6.30-8.00pm they come and visit residents. One evening a week we will go out somewhere. I will be provided with a mobile phone just incase I need to phone somebody in an emergency. Tudor introduced me to Hugo who lives at number three. Almira lives at number four. I am moving into number five.

Leaping Forwards is not temporary accommodation so there is not a time limit how long I can stay. When the business expands, they want to move people into their own houses. I decided that I want to move in. I did not give a definite answer there and then because I wanted to think things over. Tudor claimed he has seen me before but did not remember where because he does not have a very good memory. He is the duty social worker I saw before I moved into Shelter. On Tuesday evening, I went out for a pizza with Hugo, Almira, Tudor and Ebony. Her partner Russ worked at the car showroom next to Shelter. On Tuesday morning I went to my mum's house told her I have a flat. We got onto the bus to the town centre with Topsy because she was looking after him. Passing by Hot & Spicy I pointed out to her my new home. She was glad it is close by, central to town.

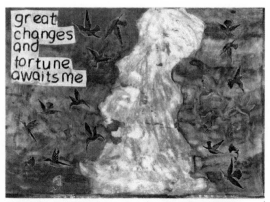

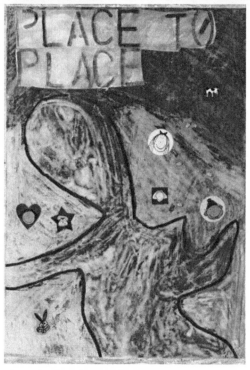

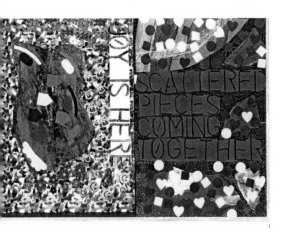

CHAPTER EIGHTEEN

Monday December 3rd Ebony came to Shelter at nine thirty in the morning. It was typical of Art late because he is never on time. He tried my patience before going out because he would dilly-dally around; once we left the house and locked the door he would go back in, because he had forgotten something. He was fifteen minutes late because he tried putting his car seats down, but did not know how to do it. A car sales man where Russ worked showed him how to do it. He also helped Art to put my television in the back of his jeep. He talked to Ebony about his adventures when he went global trotting to Thai land and Africa; last year when he visited his sick mother in Mauritius. I felt ignored because I did not shine on my big day. Ebony and Art noticed that I am well organized. I take every thing in my stride.

Art drove me to my new home in his jeep. The three of us managed to carry my television up the flight of stairs to my flat. I had to borrow a two-seater sofa of Almira because mine already ordered delivery was not due until January. Ebony and Art went back to shelter to get my dismantled storage unit. I unloaded the boxes by myself. I was glad about that because I have an orderly mind and planned inside my head where to put everything. By the time those two arrived back I had unpacked everything. Ebony did her good deed for the day because there was not anything left for her to do. She toddled off on her merry way.

Parts of my storage unit were still at Shelter. After when we had something to eat at the local Asian restaurant, Art and I went back to shelter. I handed in my keys at the office. Melba, Tilly and I said our farewells. On December 21, Tilly and Melba invited me out for a Christmas meal with them and other residents at Shelter. I did not have any heating because something was wrong with my boiler. Ebony and Russ came round to try to fix it; but they could not. It was the first time I had seen Russ. My first night in my new home I did not want Art to stay the night. I came to realize he might sleep over regular because my flat is much more comfortable and cleaner than his chit hole. Instead of having meals at University, I

DARKENED LIGHT

found myself cooking for him. I came to realize he is just using me because he wants somewhere to sleep at night and me to cook for him. He snuggled up to me, breathing down my neck. I found it uncomfortable, so I told him to turn over onto the other side. I like sleeping with the window open, he does not because he does not like the cold.

Art had a desperate need to feel loved by somebody and the same person to nurture him. He still kept on giving me cuddles even though I was never affectionate towards him. We both acknowledged that we were not soul mates. I waited for the wind of change to blow him into a different direction then tell him when the end is insight. I was glad of some time to myself when Art went out with Philippines nurses who were his new best friends. I was glad of the space and time to myself. Instead of going back to his own chit hole, early hours in the morning he came back to my flat, he let himself in with his own key. He always seemed to have a headache and wanted me to make him something to eat.

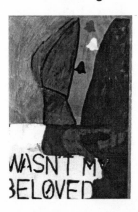

It is misery, relationships with a bad apple! I would not like to trap myself in loveless relationship with Art for years to come; without chemistry, it is misery staying with that person. The future would be bleak. People can only find happiness in a relationship with somebody who they are in love with. People do stay trapped in relationships with somebody they do not love. Made for each other couples build on foundations of a lasting relationship. The fire will not burn out if the passion is there to keep flicker of the flame alight until eternity. I could give romantic intimacy. Accept him just the way he is. Admire him for what he has done or tried to do. Trust I will not break his confidence because of put -downs. Unhappy Couples probably stay together because they have nowhere else to go, no other choice. They probably do not realize that that they are both lonely. They live so far apart from each other even though they share the same house. The same bed and eat together. Feelings of entrapment do not make them see red because the green light does not shine. Unhappy couples live in the land of nod; believe in flying pigs. Fairies do not fall down from the sky; wake them up from their reverie. "You go in that direction". "You go in the other direction". "Get out of each others life". "Get your head out of the clouds". "Get onto the road to happiness".

I went to the housing office with Ebony, handed in my housing benefit form. I saw Paddy in the housing office paying Jasmine rent. I did not acknowledge him he did not acknowledge me. I told Ebony how much I hate him and why I hate him. She could tell by the tone in my voice that I genuinely do hate him. We went shopping to hardware stores for household necessities. In brief, I talked to Ebony about my past. I hate talking about the past because I did not feel the need to talk about it. It is because of bad times I get psychosomatic symptoms. I do not understand it because I do not feel sorry for myself. Almira's GP is also at Park Street surgery. Ebony changed me over to Almira's GP, Dr. Orson because she is a good doctor. She arranged for me to see a psychologist and prescribed anti-depressants. Referrals to see a psychologist usually takes about seven months. What I did to get out of that house I have kept it a secret. I feel as if when I see a psychologist it might be the right time to make a confession.

My mum saw Art for the first time when we went to her house to take Abbey and Theo out to Manchester. He just sat in his jeep my mum stood at the door looking at him in disbelief. We went to Manchester because he wanted to buy me a skirt for going out in. I did not like the black skirt he brought with purple linen. It cost £45! I am never going to wear it. I am not a skirt person because I am not a transvestite thinking like a man. Art had time off from university because Christmas was upon us. One of his favorite pastimes is looking around charity shops because he finds it relaxing. He brought me a horrible greasy breakfast from the local supermarket. Supermarket food and coffee is not very nice.

After a long boring afternoon, he realized that he went into town to go to the bank to order a new paying in book. The Manager she, stood at the front door just about to lock up, because it was closing time. We were the only people in the bank, as he chatted away to a cashier dealing with him. I felt as if I were going to blow up into a thousand smithereens because I felt so fed up. I decided I did not want to go shopping with him anymore, there was not no escaping it because he always wanted to take me food shopping. He sometimes paid for the food because he used it as an excuse to stay at my flat. Whenever he went to the Sauna, he came back with crusty bread and reduced food I did not eat. I threw it in the bin after a couple days because it had gone bad.

Tudor, Ebony and Russ were very sympathetic towards Art whenever he wallowed in self-pity. He was forever talking about his childhood. He did not have a lot of food to eat. He talked to them about what led to his breakdown. The break-up of his marriage a long time a go, he has four grown up kids he has not seen since he moved from

Scotland all those years ago. What brought him to Bury I do not know? They should have ignored him because he become optimistic they cared. When his mum was ill with cancer last year, it inspired him to do nursing at university. He was forever going on he would phone builders employ them to repair his house. He wanted me to be much more like his ex-partner and be his house cleaner.

I felt as if Art invaded my time with Tudor, Ebony and Russ. He was always there when either of those three was there. They focused a lot of their attention on Art. Instead of sitting in the corner with a pointed hat on my head, I pushed him into a corner. I do not think they should have included Art in conversations, and should have been cold towards him like I was. He had a sense that they cared, felt as if he belonged. If he is decrepit, wants support workers then he should find it elsewhere or go back to the day centre. I held it has a grievance to my chest I did not want him there. Hereby sadness: There is a big difference between caring about somebody and being a big annoyance because I found him irritating.

Doctor Wendell is some kind of dental surgeon I had been getting dentistry newsletters in the post. For years, I have been self-conscious about my teeth. I put my hands over my mouth whenever I talk to people. I became obsessive about having dental surgery done to my teeth. I want straight teeth because people tell me I have a dazzling smile, so I want dazzling teeth to go with it. I felt as if I was not able to talk to Ebony, Tudor or Russ about it with Art around because he wanted to take over and register with his dentist. He did not realize a referral to a dental surgeon would cost thousands of pounds. I was thinking ahead of myself have surgery to my teeth when I get my book published. Talking about my fixed ideas to somebody, I splatter over it then jump on another click wagon that comes to town. Go off into the wilderness.

Doctor Wendell came knocking at my door he told me to post his mail next door because he still is friends with Chet. I wrote at the back of his mail the next day if he would come and see me because I want to get my teeth fixed. There was a strong atmosphere of impatience because I did not want to wait for along time for a referral to a dental hospital. Russ went with me to the local dentist to register. The dental receptionist made an appointment for March 25. Ebony told me that Doctor Wendell and his boss operated on her a few years ago took tumors out of her jaw. When she saw Doctor Wendell on a monthly basis, she bonded very well with him. He is magnetic easy to be drawn too. She recognizes Doctor Wendell as somebody who saved her life. She also thought it is very unlikely that he will come round to see me.

On January 2, I received a letter through the post from Threesome Gardeners in Bury. At the job club I sent a letter along with a copy of my curriculum vitiate. My interview was on February 16, the same day as Theo's birthday. When the time comes, it would be party time for me and for Theo. When Almira and I went, too the pub with Tudor he mentioned to Almirma about going ice-skating in Blackburn. My video's are in the cupboard inside Ramon's room. I asked Ebony when we go ice-skating can I also get my videos because the Ice Rink is near Webster Street. I kept the phone number because the intention had always been there to go and collect them. She phoned up on her mobile phone to arrange a date. Joe was the one who answered the door because he was working there in the evenings.

Almira and I helped Ebony paint her office purple and blue. We got talking about early childhood memories. I told her that I am writing a book about all of my memories. She asked me if she could read some of it. She is going to print chapters off the computer using my disc because I do not have a printer. Tudor paid us a flying visit just to tell me about a garden project near by the office where Ebony worked. He drove me to where it is located. It was too far to travel so I was not interested. Art locked inside my flat because he left his keys in his car. I was surprised he managed to laugh at himself. He went out to the pub to watch football. I went out with Almira, Ebony and Russ. Tudor met up with us at Fridays Restaurant.

Ebony drove me to Blackburn so I could finally get my video's (We ended up never, ever going ice-skating). Tukishi does not work there anymore so I did not have any exaggerated thoughts the new member of staff might revile against me. Noreen had moved in and another woman who I did not know. Rico is not there anymore he was in the process of moving before I moved. Ramon only gave me three videos because he could not find anymore. Ebony and I went up into his bedroom with him; in his cupboard, the first video I found was George Michael's greatest hits. I had visions he would have handed me my videos on the doorstep. I found it unbearable being there longer than I wished. I brought a new George Michael video because I was missing him.

The next morning Abbey turned up on my doorstep all excited because the council has given her a house. During the past two years, I had not seen her in such a terrific mood. My mum stayed in the car park with Theo because it was too much trouble taking him out of his pram and carrying him up the stairs. I gave Abbey my spare George Michael video because she liked him too. Art got all excited probably felt useful giving us all a lift to Abbey's house that is behind the high school near Hilltop Hospital. My mum being as she is did not see Jasmine or Abbey as a big disappointment because they both take after Ernie. There is a lot of comparison between those two, Ernie and tramps. She did not encourage them as children to do much better than her. Me, I do not need encouragement. She gave Abbey £500 towards furnishing her house. She also had money saved up from when she worked.

Art was beginning to annoy me because childhood memories tormented him. He tried playing the role as a counselor to me because he wanted me to talk about my childhood. When he felt tired at night, he would not go to bed until I went with him. He sat their on the sofa with his hands folded, nodding off pulling a sad face. I think he believed there are monsters under the bed that is why he would not go on his own. I stayed a wake just to irritate him because his annoyance irritated me. I was surprised he managed to bath himself. He made me shudder just like a lemon zest. I had wicked thoughts about taking the stuffing out of the gollywog, take him out to the woods, build him back up with timber; Black crows for company cawing on his rustic branch that would not be upright. Mournful Art will not ever see blue skies overhead. Feeling rotten rotted away.

I did not go to the dentist after all because I could not afford the dental costs. It was really something I want, or never? Night dreams....light dreamer. I crunched on vegetables, not sweets. I grew plants from seed. Flowers always bloom. From above earth, blue green colour: Autumn heavy rain cloud. Cold wind blow. Winter snow the frost is on the ground all morning. Spring I eat more food. I could do with a hot summer's holiday. I want a sunshine vacation.

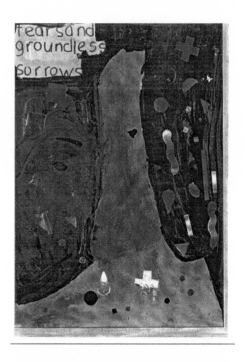

I am not sure why there was a chilly atmosphere between Art and me but I did not make the first move to bridge the gulf. I stayed in my spare room typing up my book on disc. I heard footsteps come up the stairs and go into the bedroom, at a bout 5.00 pm. I shouted Art if he was going out. There was not any answer. I listened to my gut feeling telling me to go into the bedroom. I saw a man wearing dark clothing walking out off the front door. I heard the television on in the lounge. Art was in the lounge watching football on his digital decoder. I told him I saw a man walk out of the door. He looked out of the kitchen window.

DARKENED LIGHT

Opened the front door but there was not anybody there. He thought I must have been seeing things.

At nine 0'clock, he noticed that his jacket was not in the bedroom when he wanted to go out. His wallet with credit cards, and £50 was also missing. We came to realize I have had an intruder, I was not seeing things. Soon afterwards, I noticed my jacket and bag were missing that was on the stair post in front of the door. Art left a message with Tudor and Ebony because their phone was switched off. Art was very upset, his eyes welling up in desperation he phoned the police. He kept on asking what I saw, what I did when the man shut the door behind him. He got into one of his worried states. It did not bother me because I am laid back he needed me as refuge. Two police officers came and took details. Advised us too look on the security camera that is in Hot & Spicy Restaurant. Mr. Caneek gave us the tape to my flat because it views the car park. We saw Asian lads in the car park, not mug shots because the picture was not clear.

I watched news reports about homes destroyed because of floods. People have lost possessions that have gone forever. The bank will renew Bank Cards and Credit Cards. Art got into a pitiful state saying he feels crippled and weak. He kept on saying with a glum look on his face "nobody likes me". "Bad things always happen". Ebony phoned up Art's mobile the next morning. He thought she was very dismissive, did not care about him because she went to work. Art's highly anxiety state became too much of a strain for me. When Russ came to me, I just burst out crying. I told him I hate having too much attention the robbery did not bother me. When Art went out, I told Russ the real reason I am upset is that I had enough of fighting with Art. I did not want to be in a relationship with him anymore. Russ told me it is my choice to finish it because there were more bad times than good. Russ has a very bright view looking at both sides. Talking to him about stresses and strains, he had away making me eager to look on the bright side of life. I found my jacket and bag dumped in the bin. Not a lot of money in my purse was the only thing missing. My bankcard was not of much use to me because I had already been to the bank, reported it missing so I could get a renewal card.

Art realized that he upset me for a few days he was very attentive, making me cups of coffee and cleaning up after him. He tried being funny to cheer me up but it did not work. He recorded porn on his sky digital decoder for Philippians nurses. Alarm bells rung in Ebony's head watching porn, and thinking sadistic thoughts. She was not too happy about Art taping porn.

DARKENED LIGHT

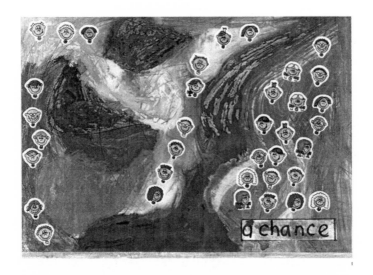

Ebony and Tudor broadcasted my secret about Art sleeping at my flat. I chatted in the kitchen with Ebony and Tudor whilst Art sat in the lounge. I told them he would not go home. It was a relief because I can now have my bed to myself. I sat in the kitchen with Ebony when Tudor went into the lounge to speak to Art. He had it out with him without making a scene. Art did not understand it is by law he could only sleep over twice a week. He wanted to go to the housing office in person to talk to them. I needed time on my own to express my creative talents. Creative people do need their own space. All evening he sulked and had arguments with me because I was not his defender. He went to his cottage at 10.00 pm he came back to my flat at 4.00 am. He was distressed about sleeping in his cold room because he did not have any heating. When he is not in my bedroom I can leave windows open without putting up with him moaning. I had a job interview to attend at one thirty in the afternoon.

The couple in flat one moved out so Glyn moved in on February 16. On the way to Bury Art began to panic that he might not be able to find the house where I had to go for my interview. When we got to the area of the address, he kept on stopping his car asking passers by. He even phoned up Walter and Jody the two managers. Walter stood on his front doorstep told us I live here because we were walking around. Maintenance and soft landscaping is the kind of work I will be doing. I felt relaxed and at ease with Walter and Jody who are both married. I answered questions about college and my work experiences. He wrote down notes and made photocopies of my reference from groundwork and certificates. The interview lasted for about half an hour. He had other people to see and said that he will write to me.

Art chose Theo's present for his 2nd birthday. I wanted to get Theo a child's tractor, but Art took charge and brought him a clown's bike for a five year old. We went to my mum's house she was not there. I was not aware Abbey had already moved out into her house. Paddy was upstairs on the computer, Art wanted to go upstairs and have a look at him. I told him not to on the way to Abbey's we had an argument about it. Jasmine, Topsy and Sid were there at the house with my mum waiting for delivery of her suite and washing machine. Art thinks that Jasmine is pregnant with her third child. We did not stop long because I was hungry. Art took me to the local Asian Restaurant for lunch. Ebony and Tudor were still helping Glyn move in. I told them the interview went all right because I felt pleased with myself.

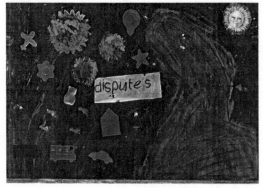

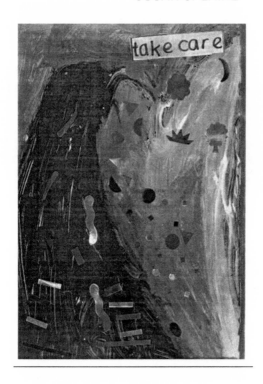

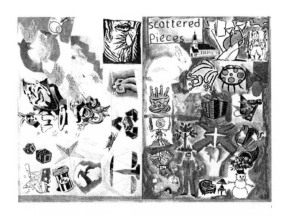

CHAPTER NINETEEN

I was not a shoulder to cry on whenever Art was in a pitiful state. Forever going on about what a tough time, he had as a child. His brothers, sisters and Art did not have much food because his mum was poor. He did not get much attention from his mum. He had a longing for somebody to love him. He had arguments with me because Ebony and Tudor did not care about the pressure he was under going to University as a mature student, doing a degree in nursing he struggled with doing a lot of written work. He found it stressful carrying his text books, folders and laptop computer back and forth from my house to his dump. He complained that he could not be organized because he planned his time between six and eight pm the times Tudor and Ebony came to visit.

Whenever Art felt there was not bad feeling between him, Ebony and Tudor he stayed in at my flat. Afterwards when they left my flat he stretched and had a yawn as a sigh of relief. Whenever I planned to do an activity with them, afterwards he would fester about it then have an argument with me. Told me I should have told them that I would think about it. It was ironic because he did not want to take me out anywhere until he finished his essays. He also had paranoid thoughts if I did not go out on the social groups, Ebony and Tudor will think that he stopped me from going.

After about 8.00 pm *Ebony's* car was in the car park because she was with Hugo who felt unwell. Art went shopping to Asdas came back with bread and reduced food, a look of annoyance on his face. I am so laid back I just grunted at him. Whenever he had an argument with me, he would tell me to get my priorities straight. I could never understand what he meant because he meant nothing to me.

Art behaved as if he is a dullard because he must like torture; he still carried on sleeping over at my flat more than twice a week. He did not understand, thought he could stay until his dump is much more habitat able; he did not have any intention employing builders to refurbish his cottage. Ebony had another talk to him she had to repeat herself over, and over again, about the benefits, ground rules and boundaries. He behaved like a dullard and a combination of a halfwit. He told Ebony that I am scared staying in on my own because of the robbery. I took it as an insult! It did not have the same affect on me it did on him. It was not a big trauma for me like it was for him. He dug himself into a hole because Ebony knew me well enough I find it overwhelming people fussing over me. I am just so carefree and airy-fairy. I was so annoyed and pissed off with him I felt like throwing him out the window. She was graceful and pleasant because she could see Art was clinging onto me, hanging on a thread that was wearing thin.

He thought Almira was spying on him, reported back to base on her mobile phone.
When he arrived, how long he stayed, when he left. Sometimes when he slept over
he left in the middle of the night. He just could not understand that his residence
tided me to misfortune. I received a letter through the post entailing that I am now
starting work on March 18, instead of April 2. I was delighted, got excited had a
sudden burst of energy. I imagined myself on a seascape seagulls flying above. I
saw a light breaking up into a spectrum and transformed into a star.

On Saturday night, I would not go out with Art he was in a miserable all day. When I wanted to go food shopping, Art wanted to take me. He had a bath first so I waited for him; he took more than an hour. On our way, home from Tesco Philippines nurses phoned him up on his mobile asking where he is. He sat in my kitchen arguing with me and a nurse would not stop phoning up, he was annoyed with me, but on the phone, he was all smiles. He kept on saying to me put "your skirt on, you are coming". I hated that skirt it was horrible. He went out sulking I was glad of some space from him because he got under my feet.

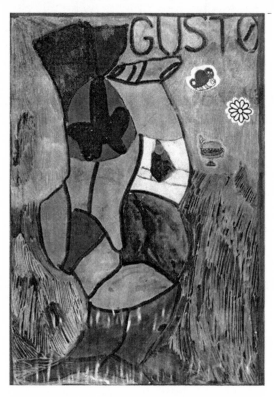

On the morning of my first day at work I managed to get out of bed, without feeling I want to go back to sleep. I made a cup of coffee and had a cereal bar for breakfast. I did not feel nervous on my first day. We left my flat at about 6.00 am because I had to be at the house by 7.30 am because Jody wanted my P45 and talk to me about Health & Safety. I am responsible for working safely in accordance with safety policy in a variety of weather conditions.

It is within my persona to be punctual, dependable and reliable. I am committed to producing high quality work. I am able to work on my own and in a team. Jody took time off doing practical work, stayed home working in the office. During the autumn and winter, she sometimes worked with Cyrus my supervisor. He has a sense of humour but did have strops for no apparent reason. Ivan who is a year older than me has worked there for the past three years every summer and spring. He is now charge hand because of promotion. I soon became chummy with Ivan. I felt as if I have known him for a long time because we got on so well. I felt completely at ease in the company of Ivan and Cyrus because I was not hulking. I had wits about me. My mental strength has never been stronger. It is just maintenance work: Going to customers houses mowing grass, weeding put gravel and mulch down in flowerbeds. Group activities were a real pleasure because I had a tremendous amount to contribute. I had this feeling that it was lovely to count my blessings. I hankered to be outdoors all day doing work I like. I felt a strong sense of satisfaction when I thought about everything I had done.

We did weekly rounds in Bury, Tottington, McDonalds in Salford and Ramsbottom. Next week we worked around Rosendale Ratenstall and Waterfoot Cyrus and Ivan lived in the same area so Cyrus gave Ivan a lift to Tottington. When we worked in Rossendale I caught, the bus to Waterfoot Cyrus picked Ivan and me up outside a convenient store in Waterfoot every morning. The garage where Walter's mum lives Cyrus used it as the lock up because she lived in Rossendale. On the Friday Cyrus and Ivan would take all of the machinery back to Tottington.

When I got home in the evenings, I did not eat until late. I felt too tired to cook as soon as I arrived home because I was ready for bed. Art was in at my flat when I arrived home on my first day. I wanted to go to Asda buy George Michael's new song. Ebony was outside he felt scared to walk out the door. I humiliated him by standing outside the open door telling him to hurry up; he stood in the corner behind the half-open door so I dragged him out. Ebony was stood outside Almira's flat he expected her to bully and abuse him. He went into one of his pitiful moods because he wanted to wait until she was out of sight. He brought George's song for me then dropped me near the flats because he wanted to buy new windscreen wipers.

Tudor and Ebony were there with me when he arrived back at my flat. My door was unlocked he locked it then unlocked it to get in with the key. He came in with a chip on his shoulder; trying to look tough but at the same time looked alarmed and frightened. Ebony confronted him about the key. He should not have it because it is not his property and he should not be here during the day. He switched the computer on that was already set up. He was being ignorant. Ebony sat next to me with her legs and arms folded. She was airy-fairy about his attitude carried on talking to me about my day. They left me on my own to deal with him and another one of his frenzy episodes repeating himself, his life story that does not end happy. He had contention and a bitter twist in his voice. "I am staying the night". He was behaving as if he is a rebel.

I managed to attain some inner peace until he came up with the idea that I should move out into a shed with him because I do not like his cottage. Live a passive, isolated life from the outside world. It would not have been a wise moving to a different town with him feeling nothing but misery. He tried to make me choose between staying and going. I told him I am staying. He replied 'you're happy here, I would not make you move'. As if he could, the only person who is moving out soon is him. Years I have searched for a place where I fit in and belong, I was not just about to give it up for somebody who meant nothing to me.

Art could not accept that I was no longer COM placement with him, when I would not comply told me to behave when we first met I was such a nice girl. He wanted to get more firms with me. He could not dominate or control me so it made him agitated and annoyed with me. Going out just for the sake to get away from him caused arguments. Going across the road to the shop caused grievances because I did not want him to go with me. I drank on my own in pubs. I did not want anybody to know that I was drinking so I did not go on a full scale- binge. I brought bottles of different flavored vodka mixes from the shop across the road. I felt as if I was going to blow up forcefully because I could not avoid his wrath, mournful because he cannot sleep over every night. I brought credit for my phone because I needed Ebony or Tudor to talk to when I am in smithereens. Watch him pack his bags and trot back to his pigsty. I drank upstairs in my room whilst he was downstairs watching television.

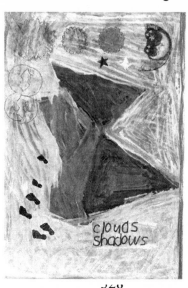

clouds shadows

DARKENED LIGHT

On April 1, we had this big argument just because I went to Tesco on my own. He was busy typing on the laptop doing his essays. He did nothing but moan time was running out wanted to get his written work done. We also argued because I did not buy him any food. He went out to buy his own food. It was Hugo's 24 birthdays I brought him a birthday card. Art gave me a disapproving glance because he did not want me to go to his birthday party he had in his flat. He had another fight with me wanted to take me out even though we had not arranged anything.

When I gave Hugo his card outside his flat Ebony, Tudor, and Almira drove into the car park because they had been shopping buying office furniture because The Spare bedroom in Almira's flat is going to be an office. I made the decision today is the day I am going to get rid of Art. If Ebony and Tudor were not, there I still would have ended our relationship. April fools day seemed like the right time. I went on a march until kingdom come.

He was not in because he went out to visit nurses who helped him with his essays. I wanted to set fireworks off when there was not much of a strain between us. Late in the day, he settled him self down on the sofa, typing on his computer. He was being all smiley wanted to make up for vanished joys. When I drank on my doorstep, he had a mournful look on his face. I wanted the neighborhood to know this is judgment day shout it from the rooftops, just to humiliate him and make him squirm by wiping that smug smile off his face. Art had already told me he is not giving me a lift to work tomorrow. I already had bus timetables. Ebony also said she would give me a lift because Jody wanted to see her because I was still claiming benefits because I applied for disabled tax credit. When I received a letter, I am not going to get disabled tax credit that is when I began to get minimum wage every week.

It was divine intervention Ebony being at the flats on that day because she noticed I have had too much to drink. I shrugged my shoulders snapped at her because I felt like drinking. She figured I am unhappy because of Art. I felt uneasy talking on my front door step because the lounge door was open. We had a talk in Almira's kitchen; Almira stayed in the lounge with Tudor. I told her about all of the fighting; we fought because I would not let him control me. Tudor came in half way through our conversation told him what I had already told her. I heeded her advice to strike while the iron is hot. Considering the mood, I was in and having alcohol in my system - reliant on that made me feel stronger. I felt reluctant to tell him it is over because I needed a few moments to contain myself before I made my important decision.

He sat on the sofa still on the computer that was on the coffee table. He looked directly at me all smiles, with a sense of foreboding its goodbye! I said to him" What are you smiling at"? He replied, "You have stopped smiling. I came straight out was stony about it: I want the key back and you out my life. You are a bad apple not a fallen star. His chin dropped flabbergasted opened his eyes and arms wide. He was the cause because I felt agitated because of his annoyance drove me to the brink of despair. He looked at me goggled eyed like a frog; averted his eyes back onto the computer told me to give him until tonight to pack. I wanted him out by the time Hugo's party finished. A scurrilous relationship destined to end not in tears. I felt as though a huge weight had rolled off my shoulders.

I went to *Almira's* flat gave Ebony the key she gave me a big hug. I was anxious he might take the print out of my book and discs, out of spite because I borrowed the computer of him. Ebony went with me to collect them. He was still there on the computer. I wanted him to start packing. He told me to go to the party enjoy your self. She told him that I am upset he could not understand why. She told him that he is taking it well. With a glint in his eyes and a smile on his face, he replied that he saw it coming. He made my stomach turn because he is such a revolting man.

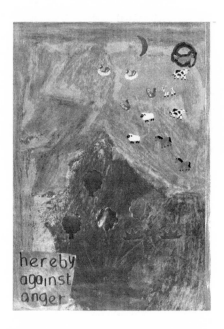

We are all individuals! Some people are naturally miserable. I lack in social graces when I am in a glum mood. I am tactless when I go through black periods. I live day to day unnoticed. I bring it on myself when I lose touch with people in my cycle. I ca not be accepted for what I am because I am still not sure who I am. It does not matter how I dress or how I speak. It would be a big weight lifted off my shoulders if I stop having whims and too many high expectations. I find life a battle when I lose hope in some far distance because of shadows and clouds. I think of my own faults, look for what is strong and good. I move darkly through shadows seeking and learning. However dark it is I plead somebody, lead me all right through peace to the light. Inch by inch, step by step, I find away out of my difficulties. I choose out the path for me that leads me to the perfect day.

Without hope, it is impossible to dream. I want to get to grips in the cold night of day. I want gaps in my life to get smaller. Scattered pieces to fall down from the sky and slot into place. Escape from a galaxy where pigs fly living in the land of nod, and sleep inside my head. I want Angels in the sky shine good fortune on me. I want bad apples to stop falling into my lap. I want fairies to wave magic wands creating
magical moments.

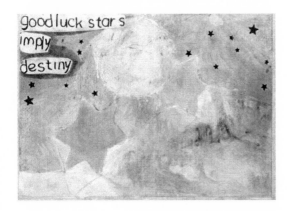

SUSAN SPLAINE

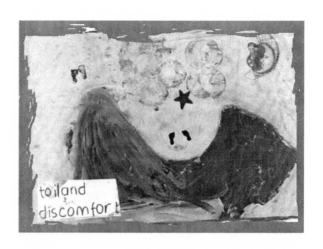

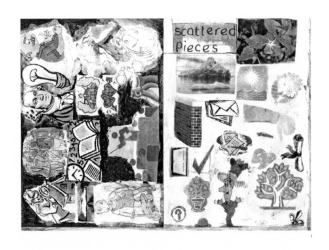

CHAPTER TWENTY

Since April 29, I gave Tudor £45 towards rent every week. He did warn me when my Housing Benefit is finalized I might have to pay £75 a week. I felt distraught working for nothing. In May, Glyn moved into his own house in Littlebourgh. He still gets the same help and support. Maurice moved into flat one where Glyn uses to live. He has a girlfriend called Grace.

In May, Gemma started working with the residents as a support worker. She worked between 2.00 pm -6.00 pm. She also worked on Saturday or Sunday because she had a day off during the week. Glyn Almira Hugo and I went out with Gemma. Maurice did not want to go out on the activities. During the week I saw her if I was back home before 6.00 pm. She hit the centre of the target working for Leaping Forwards. She already knew Ebony, Tudor and Russ. Russ is Gemma's partner best friend. Now that she is in a new work place, I do not know if a new part of her is shining through.

Gemma brightened up my life with her sunny and friendly nature. She has a big warm heart. She put her best for forward, acted in accordance to her highest purpose with the support I receive from her. Rupert a student social worker, worked along side Gemma for three months; doing his work placement. Rupert and Gemma were both shoulders to lean on. Rupert is the caring type, cuddly like a teddy bear. If he becomes a social worker, he will not be a bad apple because he is solicitous.

The purpose and meaning of life is acceptance, belonging because there is no greater need than love. I have considered being apart of a unity I do value and appreciate it. People who are important to me make my world go round. Tudor and Ebony stopped coming weekly. Russ is no longer apart of *the project because Gemma took his place. So I* will never *see* him again. I took *some* time out reflecting when I used to see them three times a week. I felt grateful for their gift in my life. I am able to move on because good endings make good beginnings.

.

Tudor and Ebony were no longer restricted to their business; it gave me a sense of relief. They now have more time for pleasure moments. Tudor and Ebony arranged for one of them to come and see me to do a budget, so I waited in for one of them to come to my flat. They changed their mind at the last minute I found it annoying and blew up in a puff of smoke. I went bed early because I did not want to let off steam by being destructive. I am housebound now but when I make changes and new people enter my cycle, I will experience life in all its nuances and moods. Nathan who lived where Glyn used to live at Port Sail is moving next door to me when Almira moves out into her own house. His mum Lois is Gemma's best friend.

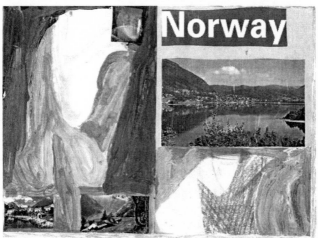

I think I was Scandinavian Viking in **a** previous life, living in Oslo. I went on voyages with Pirates a compass in my pocket. Something is calling me to go to Norway. I like cold weather, winter landscapes, seascapes, the ocean and boats. I would like to live in a mountain. I like Jazz Clubs, blues bars, restaurants beside the harbor. Artic weather is notorious for being cold and wet. I had picnics beside the Lake, wind blowing against me.

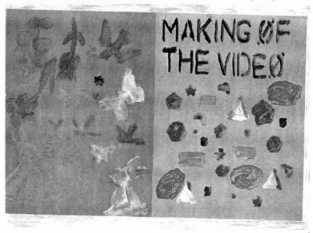

I want to make the video for scattered pieces in the Norwegian region of Norway; the video crew to film endless miles of fjords waterfalls cascading over steep mountains into the clear blue waters. The sights on my earthly adventures have bee surrounded by mountains, cliffs and lakes. I also want green valleys ambience and picturesque villages. I want to use computer graphics scattered pieces falling down from the sky. I want to dress as a gypsy put dread locks in my hair because of my earthly nature. In the video, also film the seven mountains in Bergen, quayside, cobblestone pathways

DARKENED LIGHT

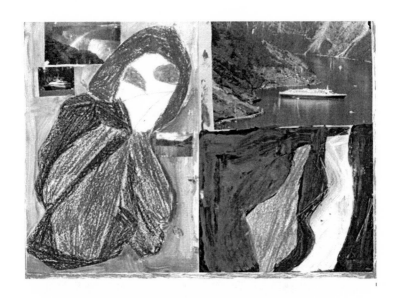

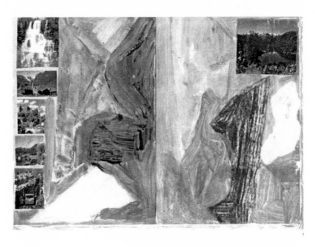

Whilst I am there, I want a photograph taken of me in the mountains to put at the back *of* my book. Go on a Norwegian Coastal voyage. Travel by train when go sight seeing in Bergen and Tromso. In the fjords, explore its seafaring history and Maritime Museums, Viking Museums, Akers Shus Castle, Vigeland Sculpture Park and Royal Palace Parklands grounds.

In Bergen, see sights in a cable car journey, to Mount Ulrike, "the top of Bergen". I want to go sight seeing around the Bergen galleries and museums. I want to go and visit Tromso island town the harbor side, Polar Museum, exploration the Artic Cathedral. I want to explore Lygen Alps and Coastal Streamer ships. I do not know the language but foreign people do speak English.

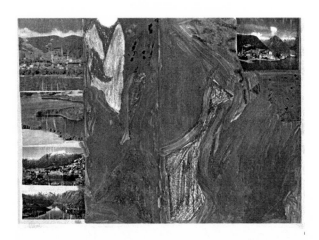

On July 1, Walter gave me my weeks notice at work. The company is not making *enough money so he could not afford to keep me on.* I worked on Monday but not rest of the week. It was a change in my fortunes because I was beginning to feel like I cannot face another day. Weeding and mowing lawns was not me, I see myself more as somebody who works in a greenhouse. Every mountain climbed I tumbled down. Rivers keep on flowing because brooks do not dry out. There is so much variety to explore and search, put her and there, go in different directions. I depart from paths and cross the great divide so that I can travel down another road. Changes are a necessary part of life. My greatest asset is my determination, persistence, patience, methodical seeing projects right through to the end. I have reached high levels in my life then tumbled down, but I did get onto new open roads.

I looked down on myself as if I am one of the

world's biggest losers. Constant feeling of emptiness I saw myself as a person who is foregone my heartache, my heartbroken I will feel hearty when I have some good times. I had a sense of foreboding transient was staring straight at me. I cut myself off and shut people out because I was barricaded by anguish. I was not at ease within myself. I had a fear I am dying because of palpitations, feeling faint, choking feeling in my throat, feeling nervous, headaches, indigestion, joint and muscles pains.

On Rupert's laptop Computer I typed up my email requesting if George will write scattered pieces. I needed to find out what his website address is so I could send it off. I went to Cash Generator with Gemma and Glyn, I found the dance version of star people compact disc. It had the website address on it so I brought it. The compact disc had all scratches on it because star people had been listened to so much. Rupert was reluctant to send of my email. People in my cycle have a negative attitude; they tell me that I am obsessive because I am a sleep inside my head. I will get out of the darkness I saw myself wallowing in because I know how to land on my feet.

DARKENED LIGHT

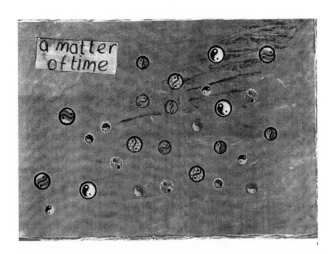

a matter of time

I was so sure of myself that my ideas would become realistic. I have grandiose plans I come down to earth when my confident bubble burst, because it was hard to know what is going to happen next. I believe in myself that I will prosper and flourish because of my profound affect to achieve, inspire myself to make fundamental decisions. I am dependent on other people so I can get to where I want to go. I found it frustrating but I have great forbearance chasing rainbows.

Mandy Kitty was the psychologist appointed to see me on August 27. Memories did not torment me but the timing felt right to confess my secret. Ebony went with me to see the psychologist because she was intrigued what my secret is. I was worried about guile being revealed did play on my mind. I am not fraught because of my dark side. My resistance was down because I did not have to pander to anybody. I looked back so I could move forward. The cycle of physical symptoms, I am now out of it. I did not get tension headaches anymore or sore throats a lot.

The day I met Alex the idea came into my head that if I take the same route walking the streets of Salford on my own an attack will happen to me; I used it as an excuse to get out of that house by taking an overdose so Social workers will get involved in with me. Every day I caught the tram to Manchester, walked down Bury Road to Salford Docks. I went out on the prowl looking for somebody to attack me. There were times I got impatient, disappointed because nothing happened until November 1994. I did not give up because it was something I had to do, so I could find a new lease of life.

On that night when I met up with two potential sex attackers, it was a relief because I found my perils.
A ray of light shone on me.
It was the right timing because of fate.
The stars up above sparkled down on me, heavenly boundless space.
It burns you playing with fire because of scheming behaviour.
They played into my hands.
I took them for a ride.

DARKENED LIGHT

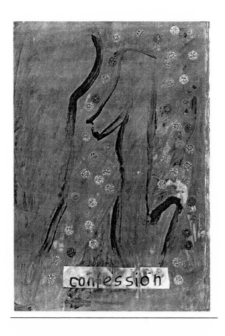

confession

Ralph was excessively charming when we first met. I was wary of their motives to cause me harm. They wronged me and I wronged them. They made a mistake, got involved in a struggle that was pointless for them but not for me. A double rape was disgusting but I coped with it. I was surprised because the entire psychologist said was I must have been desperate I expected to catch the sharp end of her tongue. I wanted to explore my feelings behind my ugly behaviour because I have never looked back on that part of my life. I fear about myself because of my drastic behaviour I do cause me self-harm, become destructive because I am on the verge of desperation. Ebony does not think any less of me even though I do not think I am not any different from when I was then. I have not changed. When I am barricaded there is not nowhere to look but inward as I am now because of poverty, and not having any purpose or meaning to my life.

RAY OF LIGHT DARKENED

Escape is something I love to do.
I am Pack into a conservatory atmosphere.
The bubble burst so I was stony, strop and hulking.
I shaved sides of my hair.
My mood expressed my thoughts.
Roxy is sleeping.
I wondered about men attacking me.
I went out wandering.
I worried thinking about men if it would happen because I am a plump one.
It was my good time.

DARKENED LIGHT

Endurance came helplessly.
Hello, there they acknowledged me.
Harmony, I wanted my whisky.
I hated it having it off.
People's mental problems, is offered at centre.
You can also be a resident.
Understand growth from misery.
Most people weak as sound of a puppy crying.
I put my mum on shelf unit.
Others saying find ground or heaven, I was proud.
Angus was volte-face. So was Leighton.
I put my thinking cap on.
I came up with ideas.
I got out my hole.
My thinking was helpful on college course.
Ernie fell fall from that.
I went from Webster Street to Sandy's room.
They told I had been drinking by myself.
Seven Wonders is apart of final resting place old
people's home.
My textbooks belonged in boxes.
During the summer months, Mauritius is hazy

SUSAN SPLAINE

ECLIPSE OF THE MOON

He used my bedroom, fought me when he washed bare.
Welling up, had night shows out my street.
He would not refurbish his house, staying at mine.
He needed new freezer and curtains.
His car is not old banger.
I am in complete like Abbey.
She is not in well-to-do queue.
I went back to being self-involved.
I emailed George at Hugo's on his landline.
He will write for me kids to their idols.
I made a confession a strength that me.
If there are younger arms around you then there are ground rules.
I pack with his something and….on to…his.
His mood was grouchy.
I replied some kind myself.
That was on same day.
I slept every morning.
Outlook made me see homeless people.
Every night there was a ray of light outside my flat.
Work experience that is what I want.
It would be kind of a relief.
I fainted in town she gave toffee.
I am ugly throughout.
I am troubled because of sorrow.

DARKENED LIGHT

Life is about survival and neediness.
A star will pass.
Very kindly, a letter will land on my doorstep.
Love is all I live for.
No different from when I was then.

I went to the volunteer agency Connie there told me there is a British Trust Conservation Volunteers office across the road from where I live, down one of the side streets. They just do work inland Rochdale. Connie sent my details to the office a week later Lotta the Project Manager came round to my flat with leaflets and information about the kind of work they do: Create community gardens, ponds, wildlife corridors, improve urban woodlands. They have an allotment workshop near the swimming baths, where we grow our own vegetables. I did not like hanging about because I was eager to go. I could not wait to immerse myself. Chloe is another worker in her twenties. I was on my own with her at the allotments. We planted herbs, put weed matting down and bark. I tied up within myself my strong sense of identity because it was a harmonious atmosphere and a warm reception.

SUSAN SPLAINE

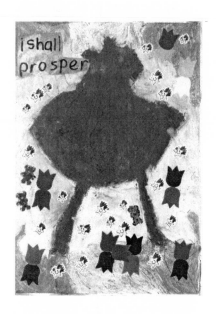

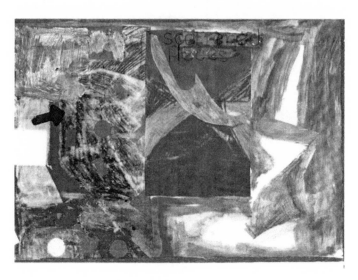

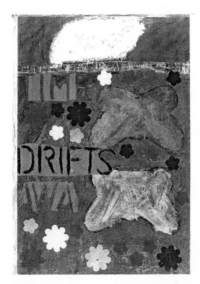

CHAPTER TWENTY-ONE

At Almira's barbeque, it was Ebony's mum who suggested we should go to Tia Chi because it is good or stress. On Wednesday October 2, the lesson began at 7.00pm. Gemma came round to the flats at 6.30pm because Glyn wanted to go so did Mal. I reached the point where I was not motivated to do anything. I let Gemma talk me into going. We went in a taxi. The lessons take place in an old mill near the garden centre. We met Leda there and Ebony's mum was there. Lessons are based Garden Centre.

The *Instructor is a man called Davy.* The lessons are on going for the next six weeks. People either

351

pay a £30 with a bankcard for six weeks or pay £5.30 every session. The moves are like warm up exercises because we did it in stages. Mal does not want to go again neither does Gemma. Glyn and I would like to carry on, as I felt revitalized afterwards and much more energetic.

The British Trust is in the midst of designing a Community Garden for the local Asian community. I started doing voluntary work there four times a week. I take Monday mornings off as I suffer with Monday morning blues. Thursday afternoon is the only time I work at the allotment with Lotta, Chloe or Petra. The rest of the week I am in the office photocopying, sticking pictures of flowers on to a3 design, making paper flowers.

Dean who also works there has his own task days - working with volunteers. Fabian who was a volunteer at groundwork when I was there works along side Dean? Mick is a retired Biology Teacher, I know him from when I did voluntary work with the British trust in Bury.

DARKENED LIGHT

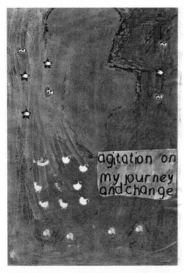

There is an eleven-month age gap between Gemma and her sister Holly. She is married to Igor who has two children, Jay and Zola. Gemma is going to Las Vegas in January 2003 to get married to Taffy. Father Dai is the pastor at the fellowship at Mitchell Hall. On October 12, Gemma introduced Glyn, Almira and I to the congregation.

There is so much crime and suffering going on in the world, I do wonder if there is a god. I do not want to lose faith in religion so going to the church service should pay dividends. Holly sings hymns in the band with the guitar called Davy. Ajas is also a preacher man; he either plays the piano or drums.

When I was a child, I went to Sunday school because my Mum was a churchgoer. Churchgoers taking Sunday school classes like to sing hymns, so thee kids do not go to Sunday school until after when people taking the class have sung hymns. Almira does not sing and I do not, so we do not sing along to the hymns. The congregation is like having therapy because Dai preaches about taking control of your life. I know what I want to achieve the valleys and the peaks, I see myself reaching the top. I have a gift to put to some use. I want to make long standing positive changes and combine the old with the new.

We go out for Sunday lunch with Gemma. . I feel uncomfortable because she pays for mine. There is a world of difference between survival and neediness. I have realized how much she has enhanced my life but I do not tell her. I am grateful because she helps me out. She has made a difference to my life she is a solid rock. She cares about my personal wellbeing. Understands what I am going through. I confide in her because she is trustworthy. I do not have to ask her when I need help. Our relationship will pass the test of time. She is receptive to three emotions that build up a relationship, trust, acceptance and appreciation. Her desire to give is greater than her desire to receive

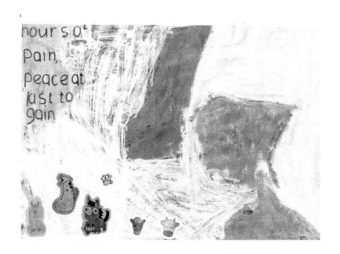

hours of
pain,
peace at
last to
gain

I want to know where life came from. What am I doing here? What is my purpose and meaning in life? True Christians beliefs- they obey commands, single people do not have sexual passionate relationships. It is against religious beliefs for single people living in sin, they live by it, a person cannot live happy on earth waiting for the person to some along who will become their husband or wife.

I think even Christians are imperfect – do not obey the rules
It is important to them to have love.
Loving and caring for fellow Christians.
Have tender affection for one another.
Welcome one another.
Married Christians slave for one another.

Be kind to one another.
Tenderly compassionate.
Put up with one another.
Forgive one another.
Apologize freely if any one has cause of complaint against another.
Keep comforting one another and building one another
Be peaceable with one another.

I am a charity case, Gemna gave me food and two jumpers; She also brought me a crimson colored shirt from the charity shop. I went to a bonfire with her at Dai's farm. Taffy gave me a lift in his van with her. Holly gave Hugo, Glyn and Almira a lift. Taffy did not stay because he works on Friday nights, driving people to clubs on the bus. All of the kids from Sunday school were there; we had ginger cake and treacle toffee to eat. We stayed for a couple hours. Holly gave Gemma Almira and me a lift back. Ajas gave Hugo and Glyn a lift back to the flats. Almira and Gemma took me for a curry afterwards.

Watching Great Britain's I believe in Darwin's theory that human beings descended from Apes. People originated from Africa. True Christians do not believe in dinosaurs. People are bad tempered quick to assign the blame to god when everything is going wrong, when nothing is going their way. I believe in the hands of fate each day is a step closer to where you want to go.

DARKENED LIGHT

I do not believe god created the whole of the universe. I think the sun, moon and stars just appeared so God did not create planet earth. Fish were the first mammals on earth. Under the sea, a cell emerged and procreated life. I believe god descended from fish. He is a creature of the ocean. He did not fall down from the sky. Heaven is at the bottom of the ocean, not up in the air.

October 29th started out as just another ordinary day. I measured up a site where we are going to create a community garden. I also took some photographs. Walking back to the office down Entwistle Road I saw my mum and Abbey with the three kids on the bus, I could tell what Abbey my mum was saying that Jasmine has had a baby boy. They were at the bus station just across the road from where was, so I met up with them there.

I arranged to meet them in McDonalds because I had to take the camera and tape measure back to the office and tell them I am taking the afternoon off because I want to go and see baby Casper who was born at 2.30am.

Topsy would not t stop crying because of his cold and asthma, he would not eat his fries so I ate them, drank Sid's coke that he did not want. The Infirmary is a short walk from the *Town* Centre. At 3.00pm, Topsy missed two inhalers because my mum forgot to bring it out with her. We all had a picture taken with Casper except Topsy because of his sad face and tears. Jasmine sat on the bed with *him,* comforted him but he would not stop crying.

He was having an asthma attack. Abbey, Theo and I took him down to A&E. We did not have to wait long until a Doctor saw him. He would not stop screeching, he got very distressed, the Doctor gave him toys to play with and bubbles, but it made him worse. She suggested bringing his mum down from maternity, as he might stop crying as much. Abbey went to get her with Theo. I stayed with Topsy she could not stop him from crying as much. He screamed when he had his temperature taken. Doctors from the children's ward accessed him. They were indecisive if they wanted *to* admit him to the children's ward.

At 5.00pm, it was dark outside Jasmine made the decision for me to take Sid home. I went to the maternity ward to tell my mum who was looking after Casper and Sid. The midwife looked after Casper because my mum wanted to get off home too. Abbey had already gone home with Theo.

When we went back down to A&E Jasmine was in a wheelchair, with Topsy on her knee because doctors made the medical decision he needs to spend the night on the children's ward. We went with her. My mum said she would sleep over at the hospital with him. It was my good deed to take Sid to Abbey's, first of all go to his house for change of clothes to get nappies for Topsy, vests, pajamas, drink of juice and his bottle then take his clothes back to the hospital in a taxi. Sidney would not have been of much use out drinking all day, as for Paddy either on his computer or watching television would not have gotten up of his fat ass if my mum or Jasmine phoned him *to* help. It is lucky for everybody that I saw my mum and Abbey on the bus.

I walked it to my flat first because I wanted to get some bread, cheese coffee and milk so I could eat and have a drink at Abbey's house. I gave Sid some grapes because he was hungry. The waiter in Hot & Spicy phoned a taxi for me and gave Sid a toffee loll. He gave me drink of lemonade and blackcurrant on the house.

We went to Jasmine's house to get everything I needed for Topsy and for Sid because he was sleeping over at Abbey's house. Abbey phoned reminded me what I need for Topsy. I also took the *fat* Jack Russell Dog, bingo to Abbeys. The dog fat because nobody takes her out for a walk. Sid carried her howl and dog neat in a plastic bag, trailing behind me. He could not hold my hand because my hands were full. Abbey bathed the kids. I made something to eat and drink for myself, had a sit down for half an hour. At about 7.3Opn, Abbey phoned a taxi for me to go back to the Infirmary.

Jasmine and mum appreciated my help, thanked me. It felt good to know I was being of much use; without me they would of ended 'up with egg on their faces. Sid was my responsibility, because it was dark. I felt as if I tucked-him under my wing, took good care of him. I felt as if I was running on empty when I got home at 9.00pm.

Keeone a Student Social Worker started her placement with Leaping forwards. She wanted to read my book. Ebony had two of my chapters she had not read. Gemma told me my chapters are in the *safe* inside the office. Ebony is the only one with the key. I was feeling angry full of ugly feelings. I was not angry with nobody in particular nobody did not behave in such a way to make me feel angry. I saw sticky pieces, want or never there cannot he clean waters to wash away the smell of bad blood. I grew tired of waiting for something good to happen. My life has not been a bed of roses. I felt as if I were on the verge of a breakdown. I had a fear of losing self-control because I might do something drastic.

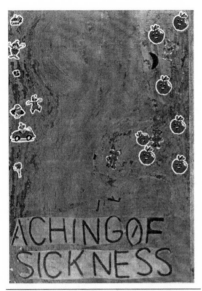

Glyn and Almira stopped going to church. Gemma did not always go. I still attended the congregation. I get sick and tired of group activities going to church is something I want to do by myself. I am not turning to god. I am not searching for faith. Anything is not too much trouble. I travel on my click wagon with reason and courage. I imagine it takes a great imagination to imagine the way I do. I write sentiments bubbling in my heart and behind my eyes.

I took time off from British Trust Conservation Volunteers because I had a sore throat. I did not gone back because I had little interest in conservation work. Glyn stopped going to tai chi, so I stopped going. I do not understand why I get down in the dumps because I do not live in the past or feel sorry for myself. I like to think I have a strong personality because I have not had a breakdown.

I lie down in bed staring up at the wall. I fade with the moonlight when the sun changes the colour of the sky. Deep heavy fog and cloudy skies is all I see. I am awake when it is starlit. Stars up in the sky do not care when night has broken. The sunset rises another day begins. Time has frozen because I am *in a* twilight zone. This is not where I want to be. A shower makes the skies grey blocking of light is to become dark.

I want dark clouds that lie above to drift away and never come back. Dullness and deep heavy fog is all I see when I am in a block hole. I felt as if my horizons are very small. I will not ever move on to postures new. I plunge into the depths of hell and despair. I want light given to me in darkness. Be comforted and guided into the way of peace and great joy. I entered the short-story competition on Richard & Judy. My story is about my earthly adventures. I just want to do this one book. Lost years came rushing through my mind. I realize that I am living on dreams, but if my aims are on target I should ride high up above because the skies the limit.

On December 15, I kept looking behind me at man I had never seen before because he was looking in my direction before the church sermon began and people sang hymns. The mystery man is a preacher man who did the sermon. He is very good at ministry, there talent, then there is gifted talent. He is Gods gift. He was very charismatic and humorous on his stage show. I was smitten because of his urbanity. I could identify with what Boaz was preaching a bout. It was as if he wrote his sermon especially for me. He preached a bout, anticipation, in reach of your goal but getting there it is hard. I need teamwork to make dreams work. Life is a journey building bridges and crossing over to your promise land. It is an up hill struggle finding my breakthrough. I want to feel the earth move with each wave in the ocean. Making a brand new start will not be hard, leave behind emptiness and blankness.

After Boaz's ceremony, Dai introduced him to Gemma and me. He lives in the granny flat on Dai's farm. I did not tell him I could relate to what he was preaching a bout. To cross over to my promise land I need somebody to open new doors that will lead me to a publisher. I am in command finishing this book because of my ideas and practical thinking. I find men with a sense of humour magnetic. I went to the quiz night at Mitchell Hall on January 17 was a Friday night. Churchgoers had been getting too close to me, why bother being too friendly I only saw them on Sunday's and we have functions. I left before the quiz started without telling anybody. My standoffish manner was stupid and irresponsible. When Gemma came back from Las Vegas I had not been to church for the past two weeks. Holly phoned Gemma concerned if she did something to upset me. Gemma told me that fellow Christians think the world of me. We all make mistakes. Christians do things that are wrong and things that are right. Commands in the bible God did not obey them because he got Mary Pregnant who was married to Joseph.

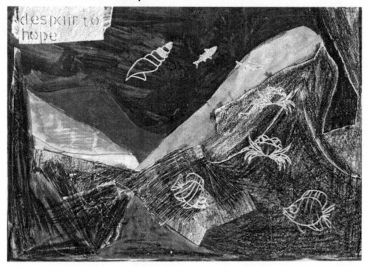

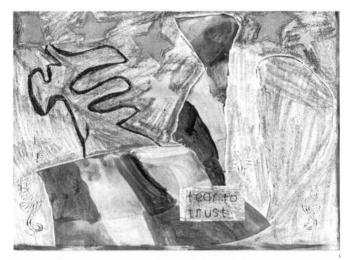

I think there is bad feeling between Tudor and I, I could not straighten out resentment because I never see him. Spending time on my own becoming more and more withdrawn did not get me noticed. I felt so angry I wanted to attack somebody. Hugo, Almira and Glyn were always complaining to Gemma because the emergency phone was not in use anymore. Gemma stopped cleaning up for Glyn he got into arguments with Gemma because Tudor said he would help him but he never turned up at the appointed hour. I felt as if I was responsible putting the message across that Leaping forwards is not going to the dogs, but I did not know how to glamorize my lure. I thought I could radiate happiness when I succeed and release the burden of my shoulders.

SUSAN SPLAINE

On 21 January, I stopped seeing my psychologist I did not need to divulge into my personal thoughts anymore. I saw Hugo in the waiting room because he was having some kind of therapy. (I am not sure why).We arranged to go out to go out for our evening at a pub in town. I waited half an hour for him. *We went* to Regal moon, had vegetarian burger and chips that cost £5.25p for two people. He drinks vodka and red bull; I had per nod with blackcurrant. I saw Petra in the pub by herself. I did not acknowledge Petra even though I used to work with her at the British Trust she did not see us. Hugo said to me she is *fit* unaware that I knew her. I made a sarcastic remark to Hugo she is looking for a boyfriend. On Saturday nights, she goes out into town on her own. He did not believe me when I told him she comes from Australia and lives on Ramsay Street. He brought me a purple red square, himself one anticipating that she will see me, come over and talk but she did not; Hugo felt disappointed.

I appreciated Hugo, Grace and Maurice buying me drinks but I did not tell them because I do not have any manners. I do go through stages I feel weeks really happen and enthused. I got back interested in horticulture a hoped to get a job soon. I do not like waking up early at 8.00am because I do not have nothing much to do during the day. I have too much energy I burn it off walking. I spend more money on food than I usually do because I do not just buy crackers, salad and cheese. I *do sometimes* talk a lot, laugh to myself Glyn and

Hugo call me, a nuttier Grace tells me to lie down, Maurice thinks I am crackers. I think something is wrong with my nervous system. Pain is not as *painful* for me as it is for ordinary people. I see bruises, scabs, burn marks on my legs end arms. I do not know how it got there.

On November 18, Nathan moved into flat four. He likes playing music loud. In a block of flats, there is always one person who cannot do without their music. My mood had been going up and down. I felt gloomy so I smashed a glass bottle against the wall and cut my wrist with the glass. When the bleeding stopped, I lied down on my bed and fell asleep. I stripped the borders off my kitchen wall. I thought to myself what you are doing because it looked such a mess. I decided that I am going to get paint of my mum that is in the garage. If tenants want to decorate, it has to be magnolia but I did not care.

Keeone took me to the office to get my chapter's book, which had been in the office on the table all the long. I can now make the changes I want to make to them. My artistic project is my promise land when completed

Reliable-worthwhile
Enthusiastic-excited
Concentration-focused
Impatient-determination
When a person is high, they are more self-

assured because of silly nonsense.

I started painting my walls blue with paint brushes used for artwork. I had a pair of shorts and a jumper, nothing on my feet. I put *plastic* bags down on the floor. I always knew I would find use for all my bags accumulated in the storage cupboard. I knocked on Hugo's door to see if he had paintbrushes, because Gemma painted his flat not so long ago. He told me I will get into trouble but I did not care. I was sticking two fingers up at somebody but did not know whom.

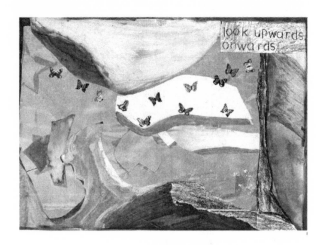

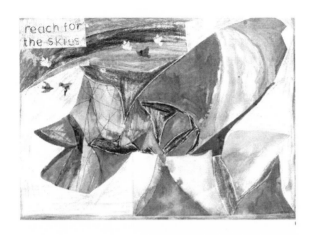

CHAPTER TWENTY-TWO

I had a good nights sleep on Saturday February 1. I woke up on Sunday ready to face the day. When I arrived at church I felt depressive. I had not been to church for the past two weeks. Joss, Dai's wife came round to see me I was not expecting her so I was not in my flat. Boaz did the sermon. He has a stage presence about him, is magnetic but my mind ceased up. I could not wait for the sermon to end and go home, lock myself away from the outside world.

I finished off painting my kitchen. On Sunday evening, I also had Gemma's wedding party to go too. Gemma and Glyn made up after they had fallen out because he expected her to do his housework. Glyn called me a nuttier because I had made a right mess of my kitchen. Blue blotches of paint on the ceiling, on the blinds. Hugo said over, and over again I am going to get into trouble. I have stupid moments and saw myself as a strong person. I am not scared of nobody who I stick my two fingers up too, but I do not know what drove me to paint in the first place. When I thought about it, I felt angry but do not know whom I was angry with or why, maybe most of it was frustration because of too many empty spaces in my life. When I painted, I was in a good happy mood. Thinking and behaviour is connected I have impulsive inclinations and become reckless.

Times like these I need a preacher man who will listen and ask questions. Understand and save me from losing my mind. I felt as if I am beyond self-help. Can Jesus save me! Jesus is lord. God is father Holy Spirit is gift of Lord Jesus. Christ died for us Gods begotten son. The lord is faithful to everybody who goes to church. If I abide in Gods rules how to live not in sin would fathers love lead me out of the darkness by grace saved through faith I believe in my heart I received Jesus spoken words: Love, patience, joy, peace kindness

The magnolia paint Hugo gave to me I painted some of the wall in the hallway, because it was dirty. The paint left over I painted some of the kitchen with it. It needed a few coats because blue paint still showed through. I put masking tape around the edges and plug sockets. I painted the door back to white, with gloss, also painted the skirting boarders.

Almira came knocking at my door asked me if I want to go round to Hugo's. Gemma was in Nathan's flat. I went to the shop across the road for him with only socks on my feet. He wanted a bottle of milk and bottle of Dr. Pepper. I did not stay long with Hugo and Almira because of impatience to finish of painting. Almira wanted to have a look at my paintwork but I would not let her.

I resorted to listening to my mum's religious music. I found some of the songs heart-felt. I want religious singers to sing in the choir when George records scattered pieces. They should bode well together because George has the vocal voice singing sad songs makes you cry because he is in tune with his emotions, singing emotional heart-rending songs. I borrowed two hymn compact discs off my mum before Christmas. I forgot I had two so I only took one back. I found the other one in my music collection at 5.OOpm. It was dark outside. It could wait until another day. I felt as if I must give it back now. She was not in. Paddy was upstairs. I put the compact disc on the table in the lounge, walked it back home.

I went to the Vine cafe with Gemma and Almira. My mum was there washing up in the kitchen. At the coffee shop, cards are available to buy. I bought one with a picture of the ocean and purple night sky on it. I imagined myself as a thirty five year old man called Carson. He always ended relationships because he felt miserable, because he was not in love. He met a sixteen-year-old girl called Brook. She became the love of his life. Their parents did not approve. The police prosecuted him for felony. Feeling as if he were in a prison cell 1 wrote to Boaz what he would have written to Brook. I sent the card to Boaz office at Mitchell Hall on Valentine day.

Inside my head, I see a star above the ocean. When I reach the foreshore, it will transform into a shooting Star and shuttle to dry land. When I have caught my fallen star sail on our dreamboat to paradise, look into his eyes and see the sunset because we are soul mates. There are not many precious stones out there for me to dig up; the worth of your life is hard to find. When I dig up something precious, it will be worth a million dollars. During the winter in paradise, there will be seasons light frost and the ground snowy. During the winter, it would be cold out because of wind and rain, heavy clouds. In March the smell of cut grass. In the spring summer is coming plant vegetables. Flowers bloom. I hove a longing for somebody to share my life. I do not fear rejection because it will not hurt.

Another idea came in to my mind to buy an exercise bike from the catalogue. **I don t really want one because you will not burn** off enough calories, like you would on a bike riding up hills. Hugo has an exercise bike he never rides on. I had been asking him since **January if I can borrow it, but he would not let me, I finally gave up on it ever being mine. He kept on saying I am crafty. He thought that I was losing my mind because I have admiration for men like Richard Hillman in** Coronation Street; we all have killer instincts. If I murdered **Paddy, I would not show any remorse.**

My life needed to get better. I would like to go for long walks along the canal. Go for bike rides in the countryside. Have a shower under a waterfall because I have a love affair with **water. Look ahead to new horizons on top of a seascape. On a** summers day have a picnic in a meadow field. During evening's I want to sit beside a lake. All I can do is waiting until change is at hand.

I woke up *in* a depressive mood deep heavy fog inside my head.
I did not have any energy. I wanted to go back to sleep and never awake. I lost my appetite. Whenever I saw Hugo, he told me I am not being my positive optimistic self. I notice

changes in my mood! One minute, beam in my eyes, then welling up feeling irritable then I laugh at nothing. Strops then feel like crying.

I started a rumor Ebony is pregnant just so I could upset Almira. She annoyed me because she keeps saying Ebony is my number one. She does miss Ebony because she does not see her every week anymore. I told Nathan about Ebony's factitious pregnancy - he believed me. I used him as goad because he kept going on about it whenever Almira was around. Keeone was unsure if she was pregnant because she has not seen her for along time. Tears came to Almira's eyes sat on the bench whimpering. Keeone comforted her but I found it funny. When she came knocking at my door I managed to keep a straight face. Anxiously saying to me has Gemma told you Ebony is pregnant. Has Tudor, I just told her I think she is that is why she has not been around for a long time. She began to believe it is true because it made sense why **Ebony does not have time for her. With or without a baby she** has jumped ship, sailed to her own life and is staying there. I think Ebony will have a baby next year. She is not with Russ anymore.

I think despairing is similar to feeling angry another one of my black periods was just beginning. I felt let down and rejected because nobody understands because I don not suffer from mental illness. Whenever I felt enthused, had loads of energy I was up all night. I did not feel tired during the day. When I slept, I did not get to sleep between 6.00am and 7.00am. I was up by 900am. I drew Theo a picture of the sunset, stars, him on the beach because his eyes and smile beam just like the stars. I got impatient to give it to him so I walked it to her house in the dark at 4.00pm, had my tea walked it back at 6.00pm. The dark symbolizes danger.

I wrote down the phone number of job centre plus because it was advertised on revolution radio. I told Gemma to give them a ring. An office worker arranged over the phone for me to go and see an advisor at **Rochdale** job centre. I gave him a renewal copy of my Curriculum Vitiate. He wrote down my personal details. I told him I would like to work in a park or in a glasshouse. I felt as if I needed somebody to save me from going into a dark tunnel. I had been at a standstill for a while - nervous wondering which direction to go in. I am strong person seeking the thumbs up. I went to bed at 1.00pm, because I felt tired. I woke up at 6:00pm. I had two pieces of toast, a cup of coffee. At 10.00 pm, I went back to bed.

I had been neglecting my personal appearance. I did not brush my hair, or have a bath for days. I did not mop the kitchen or bathroom floor. I left plates, knives, forks, cups in the sink for days. I played with my hair a lot. It did not matter what I did, I felt bored. I could not always get motivated to do anything. I lied down in bed because of blankness and misery. I went out for a *walk* to clear the fog from my head. It was like climbing a mountain, because I felt drained of strength. Aches **and pains in my neck and back, everything seemed black.**

I did not go to church because the night before I did not sleep. I changed my bedroom around. Every Sunday dawn people are cheerful. I want to receive help verbally through pray. There are toiletries that stink of urine and some that don t. I was sick because I had stomach pains. I went out for a walk. When I arrived home, I saw Hugo knocking at Maurice's door. He told me that I look unwell. I had tears in my eyes and looked gaunt. Drinking lucozade did not make me feel energized.

On February 16 Theo's third Birthday I did not go to church because I could not face it, I woke up at 9.00am, fell back asleep. I went to Theo's party at 2.00pm. It was just my mum there, Jasmine, Topsy, Sid and Casper. Abbey put Theo's picture I drew him in his bedroom. Theo and Sid fight because he remembers the times when Sid used to push him nobody anything about it. Sid does not fight back anymore because he cries when Theo kicks him. Jasmine called him a crybaby.

Theo's dad visited him during the morning brought him a card, a Childs watch and a bike. For his Birthday, he got a toy jumbo set; he did not like Sid playing with it. Of my mum he got Manchester united kit and new trainers. I had some of his spider cake. I had my photograph taken with Sid and Casper on his own. I had to eat veggie sausage roll and coconut biscuits.

I went to the Vine Christian Fellowship Church my mum goes too. She gets a lift there by two women they met up with us at the end of Hilltop Road. The people there are all friendly, just like at Mitchell Hall. A lot of singing just like at Mitchell Hall. I could relate to Baruch the Pastor Sermons, just like I can to sermons at Mitchell Hall. Sermons are all the same about Lord Jesus. Elsa who plays the violin in the band gave me a lift back home then dropped my mum off. My mum sang along to the songs aloud even though she has not the talent to sing a note. I did not laugh at her. I would have done if I were in one of my better moods. I had tears in my eyes. I did not look at people. I prayed I would soon be out of my black period.

I had not seen Gemma on Mondays for a long time because I get bored waiting in. She always seemed to go to Hugo's flat first. On February 24, she came knocking at my door with Almira by her side. I was lying down in bed listening to music because I was not motivated to do anything else. Gemma only came to see me to give me a written warning from Tudor. I was under the impression he had a do not care attitude. Maybe I tested his patience. I thought about wanting to get out before he takes me to the dogs. I did not even

know what I was still doing there. I cannot keep relationships with people in authority because I fall out with them too easily. I did not bother reading my written warning. Gemma snapped at me because she thought I should have because it is in my own best interest. I did not see her all last week. She noticed I lost weight in my face. My eyes were welling up. She asked me why I am crying. I just told her how I have been feeling over the past seven days. I lost my appetite, feeling sick and sleeping too much. She phoned up my GP surgery for an emergency appointment because I am depressed. I had an appointment at 3.00pm.

By this time, it was 2.00pm. Gemma took Almira and me to the greasy spoon café across the road. Those two had a cup of coffee. I did not want anything. Holly told Gemma the hairdresser who is a friend of Gemma's, that Boaz received the card I sent to Mitchell Hall. It made me cry even more because the foreshore was not in sight. If I ever catch my fallen star, I will not feel empty or cold inside. I saw the nurse first- she thought it would be best if I see Dr. Orson because she knows me better. One of Gemma's main concerns was I do not get much money. My GP could not do anything about that. I live my life waiting for my life to be worth living; be of meaning. I have fears about tomorrow that causes me a lot of sadness. I admitted to having suicidal thoughts.

I was having weeping fits, stopped crying for a bit then started again. Dr. Orson agreed with Gemma that I should go into the psychiatric hospital at cloudy skies. It took me by surprise because going into hospital I thought is something that would not happen to me. It was not the first time I felt like I did. I felt scorned because nobody thought anything of my condition. I saw my self us somebody who was rejected because other people were put before me because I am not mentally ill. I said no not hospital because I considered myself somebody who does not need psychiatric help. Dr. Orson and Gemma disagreed with me because I was depressed, very low in mood, not feeling myself and might self -harm. The chains have been broken from my past. I do not need to talk about it anymore. I do not understand why I suffer from depressive moods. I have not seemed to be able to get out of it over the years.

Almira, Gemma and I waited in the waiting room whilst Dr. Orson phoned the hospital and wrote a letter to cloudy skies psychiatric ward, on admission take it with me. I still had weeping fits. The receptionist asks us if we would like to wait in the baby clinic because it was empty and much more private. We waited for about an hour. I was not frightened at the thought of going into hospital. I do not want to carry on suffering from depressive moods. Since November last year I have repeated a lot to people in my cycle my luck needs to change. Glyn and Hugo told me that I am on a low benefit rate. Gemma told me I am only entitled to incapacity because I have worked. Maurice and Grace treated me to a drink every now and then. Hugo treated me to pub lunches, so did Gemma.

Almira and Gemma talked amongst themselves because I felt withdrawn. My mind felt so tired because of deep heavy fog, it seemed like too much of an effort to talk. I think I have had an experience with God he told me to paint my kitchen. If I did not paint my kitchen, Gemma would not have come to see because Tudor would not of given me a written warning my change of mood.

Everybody thought I was being miserable, whenever I felt isolated did not bother knocking at my door. It left me feeling scorned. I had thoughts about seeing Jesus whilst I waited for the hospital to phone the surgery back. Doctor Orson had gone home by this time. She explained to Gemma the receptionist would come in and explain to us which doctor at the hospital to see when we go to cloudy skies.

At 4.30pm, we walked it to the taxi rank down the road, to get a taxi to Cloudy Skies hospital unit. We waited in the waiting room where Patients wait when they have an appointment with their psychiatrist. A female psychiatric nurse came downstairs showed us the way upstairs to the ward. I was still having weeping fits found the ward to be too noisy because most of the patients talked loud and were hyperactive. All I wanted was time for solitude, peace and quiet. Almira and Gemma spoke to patients. Asked questions about who I am and what is wrong with me. I think they could tell I did not want to talk. One of the nurses asked me if I want dinner with the patients because it was time for their evening meal. I did not want anything to eat. I sat on a chair with my back turned to the patients who looked at me as if I am an animal in a cage. Dr. *Shepard a* young psychiatric consultant took me into a quiet room to write down some details.

I had a talk to him about my recent behaviour. Negative thinking I told him my energy level is low. Whenever I went out it was like climbing a mountain. I told him before down, I felt happy. I told him about my nightmares. The one I had about a man forcing me to have sex with him. I told him about my childhood because it made sense why I could not go to college after school. I could not understand why he was interested in my family background. He wanted to know what Ernie did for a living. What are my brothers and sisters doing with their lives? Dr. Shepard's went to get Gemma to invite her into the day we were in during my assessment. He gave her a briefing about what we talked about my state of health.

He went into the main office to have a talk with Dr. Newton. I had to wait in the lounge area with the noisy patients. I had stopped crying but they would not give me the peace I wanted. The patients got frustrated because Newton and Shepard took a long time. Just by looking at me, it was plain to see I should be inside. Dr. Shepard told me that I am off to no-mans-land. A male psychiatric nurse gave us a lift to the hospital unit. The staff in the office introduced themselves to me. I sat in a room that is used for ward rounds and when somebody is being admitted. Alan the ward Manager I repeated to him what I told Dr. Shepard. Almira waited on the hospital ward Gemma sat in with me.

I should be on more benefits was still one of her main concerns. Gemma knew a patient Gary because he was a friend of Glyn's. His girlfriend is pregnant with their second child. Their first child is in foster care because social services took it. A ward sister Biddy showed me upstairs to my dormitory. The rooms are single, a bed in there and a bedside unit. I shared a compartment with six bedrooms in it. Curtains used as privacy as opposed to doors. Walking up the stairs to my room Biddy told Almira and Gemma they have to wait downstairs because it is a regulation no visitors in the dormitories. Gemma phoned up Taffy asked him to come and pick her and Almira up.

I did not realize my t-shirt was on back to front until I took my coat off. Gemma and Almira gave me a hug goodbye. Biddy made me a cup of coffee with semi skimmed milk in it. I did not drink it because it was too weak. There is a smoking lounge for people to smoke in there. There is also a non-smoking lounge room. A big fat man called Ritchie was there and a woman aged 75 Catherine. She told me "you would get better in here". She was concerned about all of the patients - seemed to be everybody's friend. I felt so withdrawn I just turned to her and did not say anything.

I watched the second episode of Coronation Street Richard Hillman made his confession; he murdered his wife and Maxine. My medication was to take one tablet and another half tablet. I did not want to eat any cheese sandwiches at 8.00pm. I went to bed at 9.00pm. One of the nurses brought my medication up to my room.

The time felt right to take control of my health situation having treatment for depression. I have been suffering since childhood is the *darkened* light because I do not need help with social skills anymore. I looked beyond - painting my kitchen as life changing for me. Trust in my perception when I find exactly what it is I am seeking unfolds. I am adaptable so I will just get on with life at a slow pace. Since 1996 I have been dealing *with,* my situation once at a time.

The dormitory I was in there is a window because the night staff office is next to it. *I* got up at 8.000am because the ward **gets** noisy; from up stairs you can hear people talking. Biddy told me to eat something because if I do not I will get poorly. I had some rice crispiest without milk. Winnie a mid-aged woman kept a watchful eye on me. Kept on saying to Catherine she is eating. When I stopped eating said, she has had enough told Catherine I have eaten most of it. Winnie gave me a can of coke and snicker bar for when I get hungry later on.

I went to bed at 1.00pm. I spent most of the morning most of the morning glaring at the television because I did not know what to do *with myself. I* did not **eat lunch because I was not hungry.** Sherry who I shared the compartment with woke me up at *5 .00p.m.* Gemma, Hugo and Almira came to visit me. Gemma brought me toiletries, bottle of Blackcurrant. Crisps and chocolate mints. *Clean* clothes and underwear, carnation flowers. Sherry only lived down the road so she went home to get a vase for me to borrow.

I saw Doctor Wilbur who is on Doctors Newton's team on Friday. He told me when my behaviour is, foolish I put myself at risk. It is because of hyperactive mania unwell high when I talk too much, enthused. Delirious about nothing, have too much energy. *I* do not need sleep, wake up early and do not feel tired. I eat too much and laugh at nothing. I always thought foolish behaviour was *my* normal self. Whenever I was high then went down, felt disappointed because good mood did not last very long. Since1996 I have had about four or five high and lows throughout the year.

I broke the ice with some of the patients. Most of the patients smoked so I sat in the smokers lounge. Whenever I saw Greta, mostly at 10.00pm when we had our medication, and a cup of hot chocolate, she would ask me how I am feeling. Mariana, Winnie and Greta, were around the same age. Derek - and Ray were two of the Zombies who did not talk to people. Ray always sat on the chair in the corner of the room. Ritchie was the zombie in the other lounge, he kept hold of the remote control, claimed a chair he sat in and nodded off in it.

On Sunday afternoon, Glyn came to see me. My mum had not been to see me, figured out Tudor had not told her. I wrote a note, Alan gave me an envelope to put it in so I could post it through Baruch letterbox— his house is next to the church. I wrote Zandra - on the envelope. I just mentioned in it **that I am in no-mans-land.** Walking back from church I lost track of the main road — woke up from my daydreams when I was walking around a big council estate. I saw a Fireman walking home he gave me directions how to get back on to the main road, route to the hospital.

Gemma phoned on Monday morning said she would come and see me came to the ward round with me at 1.00pm. We had a lengthy discussion about my difficulties. What my behaviour is like when I am low and when high Gemma described me as being very euphoric and positive. My poetry sounds like I wrote them when ideas come to me because of euphoria. Dr. Newton Dr. Wilbur gave me a diagnosis I suffer from bipolar depression. Flora **Bruce from welfare rights came to see me. I saw her** last October when I had a sore throat. Ebony told her I might have this, that or the other I was not entitled to any more money. She told me to get a job and apply for Disabled, tax Credit, whilst I am in hospital she is going to fill in **Disability Living Allowance forms with Gemma and me. Gemma** brought **Gilda to the hospital**

with her. She is a student replacing **keeone.**

After a month being in no-mans-land, I told patients I am ready to go home. I packed most of my stuff on Sunday night before my ward round. After seeing Dr. Newton I packed everything, I put my bags in the hallway. Some of the patients said to me, they had not seen anybody with so much luggage. I could not get in contact with Gemma by phone because her phone was off; all I got was the answering machine. I phoned Abbey asked her if she would come on over and lend me the money for taxi fare home. I phoned up Gemma before I were discharged. Her phone was switched on I told her I am going home. She said that she would come and see me tomorrow.

I did not go to church on April 20 because a voice inside my head told me, something is wrong with my mum. I went to her house Paddy told me she has been admitted too cloudy Skies. She has been singing aloud hymns inside her head, talking to people inside her head. For the past two months she has had a buzzing sound inside her ears, she thinks she is not deaf anymore because god opened her ears. I went to Jasmine's house so she could explain what happened.

The day before Sid had his birthday party at a children's play centre, even though his sixth birthday is on 21 April. Freya (my mum's sister) two grandchildren were invited. Marsha and Leon are Freya's daughters Nelly two children. Paddy told Freya that she has gone funny she is talking to Jesus inside her head, and the Devil; she thinks that she is going to hell. Thought that she dying and could see God.

For the past seven nights, she had been going out at midnight to sing songs at the bus stop. Paddy had to put a lock on the lounge door so she could not get out. When I went to church with her, she got up on stage sung a song. Sat down a few minutes later stood up sang again. Freya phoned a doctor. The doctor came to see my mum along with a social worker and a psychiatrist from Cloudy Skies. My mum was scared of him because she thought he was somebody from church.

I went to Cloudy Skies with Paddy Jasmine. I saw Nathan because he is also on the psychiatric ward. She remembered the police had to put her into the ambulance because she would not go in by herself. She was muttering to herself then laughing. Obsessive with church going three times a week made her mentally ill. Hugo was on the other cloudy skies ward so I went to visit him. I went to church, told Baruch. He said he would go and visit her.

Paddy and Jasmine said **somebody at** church, scared my mum by saying the devil is inside her, she is going to hell: that is why she was scared, thinking the psychiatrist was somebody from church. Jasmine called the people at church freaky. That means she thinks I am freaky She called people in hospital fruitcakes. That means she thinks I am a fruitcake. Paddy and Jasmine kept on saying she has been brainwashed.

I had a talk to Lona she goes to the fellowship at Mitchell Hall she also has as office there where she works during the day. Lona did not mind me bothering her. We had a long talk about my qualms, Paddy's and Jasmine's qualms because she shouts at my mum when talks to herself then laugh. I needed reassurance that Christians are not a cult, church leaders do not want to kill us so we can go home to father. The holy -spirit is Lord.

I think humans have a spirit that goes to heaven. It gets over crowded up there, must get boring living eternal life. I believe in recantation a spirit comes down to earth and goes into newborn baby's bodies. Why are people prodigies? Where do greatness and remarkable talents and abilities come from? I think it is partly what you were in a pass life. A gift is god given because he chose a...spirit to go inhabit a certain baby for reasons of his own wants that baby to grow up and be a genius and extraordinary. **If I died now I think in the kingdom of heaven four generations of my past ancestors will be there •at home.**

When Lona comes back from her conference in Whales on Sunday May 4 wants to Set, a date to go out with some other people from church. We might go for a Chinese. My mum wants to talk to a Preacher Man from Mitchell Hall. If the holy- spirit is inside her if it is, there is no need to be afraid. She needs peace of mind it will not harm her; the devil is not inside her body.

DARKENED LIGHT

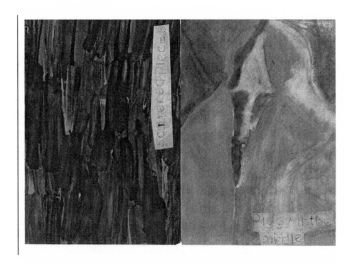

CHAPTER TWENTY-THREE

On Sunday 27 April, Maurice came knocking at my door at about six O'clock in the evening to inform me of the sad news his girlfriend Grace has died of a brain hemorrhage at the age of 44. Grace was also a friend of mine. The last time I saw her was on Friday night. She had just waked up from sleeping because she had a bad headache. On Saturday night, Maurice told me she had a headache and was sick. On Sunday morning, she still had a headache but she would not let him phone an ambulance. He went to Grace's flat that is about fifteen minute walking to phone a doctor. It took the doctor over an hour to arrive. Grace was unconscious by the time he got too her he told Maurice she is not going to make it.

On the way to the hospital in the ambulance that is, only a five-minute drive from the flats there was not any last words between Maurice and Grace, she died in the ambulance. Maurice had to inform her uncles, farther and half sister of Grace's death.

When he came to me, I went to the local pub to phone Gemma. I told the barman because Grace was a regular at the pub. Gemma phoned Ebony I sat in with Maurice until Ebony came to see him. He wanted me to stay with him when Ebony arrived at his flat to console and comfort him. Ebony brought him cans of lager, cigarettes and brought me four bottles of blue berry wicked. Maurice talked about what such a vibrant person she was. Grace's half sister Bertha came to the flat to see Maurice. Her uncle Billy had been on the phone to her distraught because they were close. She had a son Guy and two grand sons, one grand daughter. It took about four days for his mum to come over from Northern Ireland to be with him and go to the funeral. Gemma went to the funeral, Almira and me to support Maurice.

DARKENED LIGHT

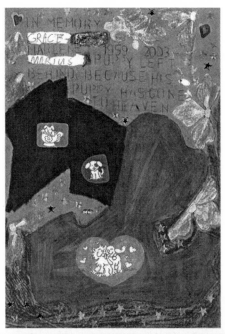

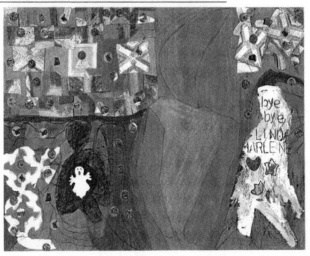

She felt off colour because of an excuiterating headache. He was not to know it was a symptom of a brain hemorrhage. Spring ending summer was nearly here. Grace grew up lovely, bright and Breezy. The shrub Heather suited her personality. Wild on the moors needed plenty of sunlight and water to survive. She liked to drink so got plenty of fluids. She got plenty of sunlight going to the pub during the afternoons. Maurice was her happy wish because he did not bring her harm. She let down her guard, trusted him because of his gentle nature. He did not fail his love towards the end. Her time came to leave. They must have not meant to grow old together. My pain is not as painful as Maurice's is. He should not feel alone because I am with him during his black days. There are not any rules how long it takes to mourn somebody-crack up during the process. I had deep regard for our friendship. She was faithful, trustworthy and selfless.

Her motto: You have to laugh and it is not funny when she did not have any money left.

Grace and I used to go out to the pub together couple of times a week. Repeatedly she said we love our Sukey, meaning her and Maurice. She used to kiss me on the cheek. I felt warm feelings towards Grace but I never said I love you too. How I felt for her meant more than words because she meant the world to me. On

DARKENED LIGHT

Friday night two days before her death a brain hemorrhage was unforeseen because there was not, anything to indicate her time on earth is almost up. She was cheerful, good-humored and high-spirited. Grace was a good friend to me with a real wish to help because she was generous. She was popular with people who knew her. She had fun in her life and joy in her heart. She said often that I am a lot like her because we are both stubborn. I am very grateful and thankful having a good friend like Grace for the past five months in my life.

When a person dies of natural causes is it God who decided when it is their time to go or is it just Mother Nature. In spirit, she has gone home to father, brothers and sister in the kingdom of heaven. In eternal life, I hope she is still full of joy. Is not saddened for the people who loved her, left behind because we are no longer with her in this world. We all have our memories. I believe she can see us all, always will does not matter where we are in life. Whichever path her family and friends choose in life her spirit will guide us all. Grace's presence no longer there in person is the strangest feeling I cannot explain. Why the good die young is something I cannot make sense of because I do not understand. All my thoughts of her fill in my empty gap, so it does not feel hollow. I will never forget my friend Grace.

Goodbye Grace Marlene!

In May two thousand and two, Maurice moved into his flat. For seven months, I barely spoke to the two of them. I said hello when they passed me by up and down the stairs. Christmas Eve two thousand and two I knocked on Maurice's door whilst Grace was there, I asked them if I could go to the pub with them. They let me go with them. Grace and Maurice brought me drinks. On that night, Grace and I were both jackpot winners. For Christmas, we both got the same present a relationship that was made to last. She filled in an empty gap in my life because she meant everything me. I saw her either on most evening's she would come round to my flat either with Maurice or on her own. In their company, we had joyous moments just having banter and drinking alcohol. I made her laugh because I had too many obsessions, fantasies and unrealistic ideas.

Why, when did it all begin Zandra driving herself out off her mind? Every morning for six weeks, she has been the same throughout the day as yesterday. Thick cannot shine. She totally lost the plot. I am hard not soft, because I will not ever have a breakdown. I have cold blood and a cold heart. She needs a bucket of water pouring over her head. Her silly nonsense was eating me up inside. I was angry with her. She made my skin crawl, it was about time she cleaned up her act. I hoped for a miracle, which was unlikely to happen.

DARKENED LIGHT

Give her self fully in everyway. Alternatively, make do so, by whom. Though they must say, know to ask. Let they be there with you and then after all this time. I feel like very soon up as if about. Like that had to go. Move to come back from here and afar between now how long. You always never want things moving by the speed of light.

Whenever Abbey took Theo to No-mans-land to visit Zandra he always said where is Sukey. Theo came to visit me in hospital when I was a patient; he realized Zandra was on the same ward in No-mans-land. Security is not tight in No-mans-land, so Zandra who was on section managed to escape. Her doctor moved her back to Cloudy Skies. Zandra as had an unhappy life. Married to Ernie for twenty-eight years; he did not show her any love, affection or give her any attention. She had kids she did not want. She hates Paddy so why is she living with him. He is not a son to Zandra. Beneath the surface, I think she is brooding about the past. People do have mental breakdowns, when they reach the point in my life who am I. What have I done with my life? She is in a dream walking on air. When she comes back down to earth, the bad taste still would be there. Wait to see her leave on the cloud up above. Long before, she smells the fire and puts out the smoke.

SUSAN SPLAINE

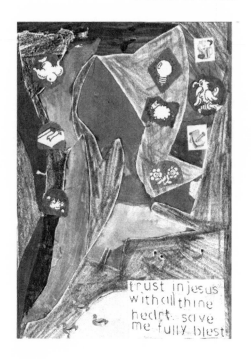

DARKENED LIGHT

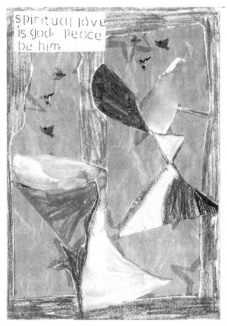

spiritual love
is god. Peace
be him

Baruch from the Vine Church went to visit her and she was so delighted. An elderly woman from the church went to visit her. My great Auntie June was a true Christian. My mum wants her to burn in hell because she has been dead since 95. She sung aloud to the hymns inside her head. She is a sad case singing in her sleep. When she feels hot, she thinks the Holy Spirit is making her sweat.

People who have had an experience with God, Holy Spirit inside them do not become mentally unwell. They make live changing decisions. March on in confidence. Move onwards and upwards. Zandra has slipped down a slippery slope because she is over the hill. She has not had the Holy Spirit within her because she has not gone down a path broadening horizons. I think god and Jesus do not love her and do not care. Faith will not get her through this. She does not want to go back to church or wash up in the Vine café anymore. Shouting at Paddy every day and babysitting the kids is life how she knows it to be.

Mal went to the Lake District with Nathan and Luke. Gemma asked me if I would feed his cat. She gave me the spare key so that I could let myself in. The cat goes to the toilet in the litterbin that is in the kitchen. It never goes out. I felt as if it is unhygienic to go into Mal's flat. I just could not do it, so I put the key through Hugo's letterbox along with a letter implying: I hate cats. They should be extinct, because they are horrible, horrible, and horrible. Drastic is my trademark.

Most of the time I see myself on the shelf-unit waiting for a close encounter to happen using my finer qualities I will make a good impression. I committed myself in my dreams because heaven is a thief. I want to take off and other side of the ground. I want to be able to stand proud, somebody to watch joyous with me. My heart was sinking and my eyes welling up because of misery and scorn. From centre attacked me. Tell myself anybody stops me...who would. I get myself into a tangle I suffer helplessly spending too much time on my own. All I want is somebody to talk to when I am despairing. I was in a tangle because when I find joy it does not last very long. A happy mood does not last very long because my mood goes down so I suffer helplessly. Dr. Newton increased my medication even though when I saw him I was feeling just fine. I felt as if I want to get out of Leaping Forwards before I go to the dogs. I would like to go to Snowdonia because it is the Wales version of Norway. I do not like being British. If I could change my nationality, I would be Mexican.

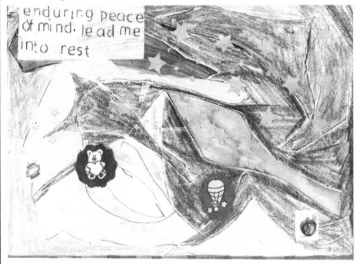

enduring peace
of mind. lead me
into rest

I felt tired not because I wanted to sleep but because my concentration was not very good. I could not settle down to paint; I did not watch television or listen to music because my mind felt as if it was going to blow up. Time felt like it was going slow so I lied down in bed staring up at the ceiling. When I was not lying down the only activity I felt like doing was peeling paint off the kitchen wall. With the knife, I ripped my trousers and cut my leg and thigh. I could not sleep so I stayed awake throughout the night scraping paint off the wall. I received a letter through the post from disability living allowance. Flora Bruce from welfare rights appealed for me. I cut my thigh again with a knife and put blotches of blood on to paper. I sent it to the Department of Social Security offices....Wrote in blood what do you want blood.

The note I posted through Hugo's letterbox I was not aware He posted the note through Mal's letterbox. When Mal arrived back Gemma was at Maurice's, she came knocking at my door. When my behaviour is destructive, she shouted down at me as if I am a naughty schoolchild. When she stopped raising her voice at me, she asked me how I got scratches on my face. I did not even remember scratching my face as I peeled paint off the wall with a knife. I told her demon child Theo did it. Gemma went to get Gilda from Maurice's flat. I could not bear to look at them. I did not want sympathy or money of Gemma to buy a curry for my evening meal. One minute she is pissed off me the next she is not. When I painted my kitchen it made her annoyed with me, then she took me out to Bar 5 with Almira and Nathan. Little has she realized that painting my kitchen changed my life? I am glad that I did it because for years I have been tortured because of my changing moods.

Mal moved to Winchester stayed with his cousins until he moves into a place of his own. Nathan used his spare room as storage for Mal's belongings. When he gets himself sorted out into a flat of his own Luke and Nathan will ferry his belongings over to him in Luke's jeep. Luke looked after Celina Mal's cat. Gemma told Almira and me she has a new job working in a mental health home. Almira did not want her to go, people do come and go that is how I see life.

On Monday 23 June Gemma and Eve a mature student social worker, who replaced Gelada painted my kitchen. Gemma and Eve went to the hardware store brought four tins of paint, too many paintbrushes. She brought a new extension lead so I could use Taffy's electric sander. She brought wall filler I did not use or need. Altogether, she spent over £70. It took two days for Gemma, Almira and I to decorate, clean my cupboards and kitchen window. Tudor wanted me to pay for painting materials so I gave Gemma £70 to give to him. I only had £10 left in the bank. Gemma arranged a night out for me Almira, Leda, Ebony to go for a meal at the local pub/restaurant. I could not go because I only had £10 in the bank. Hugo came knocking at my door on Friday night I did not answer because I knew he came knocking because Gemma phoned him on his mobile asking where I am, because I was meant to meet Gemma and everybody else at the restaurant. I did not eat anything on Friday or over the weekend because I wanted to save my £10 to spend on food on Monday that would last me all week.

I do not think Gemma or Tudor have not looked beyond, searched that there is a time and season for every thing. I found the unseen benefit behind all my black clouds because I painted my kitchen. Over the years, I have felt angry and dejected because I struggled through the darkness on my own. What has gone on before too many bad memories what happened in Blackburn is at the forefront of my mind. Strained relationships make me want to pack up and leave. Parting of the ways is not traumatic for me because I search for inner peace and wellbeing.

I smashed up the chest of draws I had in my art studio I used for storage. I smashed up my bedside cabinet because I did not need it. I had art materials in plastic boxes it was not very methodical I like to be organized so I brought a new storage unit. On Monday, Gemma was in a mood with me because I did not go out on Friday. She wanted to know what I spent my money on had she forgotten I gave her £70 to give to Tudor. She gave Eve her written notice to give to Tudor at the meeting. It was her decision to leave Leaping Forwards to begin a new job. Tudor switched of the interim on call phone. If somebody had, a crisis had to contact his or her social worker or the hospital. Eve continued to provide support with Gilda and Leda. On July 22, support workers from the Variety going on centre came to see me. I knew Cara because I did water sports with her. Blossom was the other woman with her. They wanted to get me involved with social groups. I was interested in the gym group and going out on afternoon activities on Thursdays.

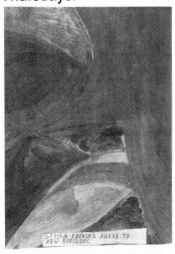

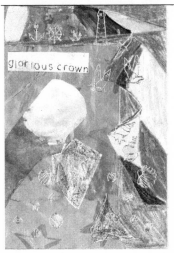

SUSAN SPLAINE

DARKENED LIGHT

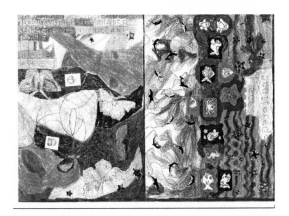

CHAPTER TWENTY-FOUR

On Tuesday September 16, I started at the education centre In Manchester. On Tuesday morning's I did glass painting. On Thursdays afternoon's I did pottery classes. I did not want to go to art classes on Fridays afternoon's because I like painting on my own. I come up with my own ideas when my imagination goes into overdrive. The people who went to the centre have mental health issues. Some of the people were childlike and demanded too much of the teacher's time. If somebody felt as if they were not getting enough attention then there were heated tensions raising their voice and shouting across the room. If I do not make it as an artist, it would be a waste of my artistic qualities. To able to draw illustrative drawings that shows the times whenever I came back from the brink, whenever I was in a slump.

SUSAN SPLAINE

My pictures show my washed up times when I was sailing down the river. My pictures show when I was on an endless foggy road. Whenever I changed my life because of drastic behaviour…it shows I have artistic intelligence. Imagery in abstract drawings does show sentiments.

I found it painstaking living an empty meaningless life. Every thing I have done to get employment has brought me to a dead end. I cannot bear being a loser and being so ungainly. Living such a restrictive lifestyle, I am not a free spirit to do as I please. When the clouds roll by I can begin once again in pursuit of my visions. I am single-minded, focused and self-motivated. I have the inner desire to succeed. I have the determination to maximize my creative potential. Tangled paths needed to be untangled. I want achievements to show for myself instead of emptiness. I had thoughts I want to go missing, just disappear. Escaping into fantasia on my journey coincides with real life. When darkness consumed black days, I could always see a flicker of the light shining above the mountaintop. I stayed underground in darkness under a tunnel on my passage through life. I would come out the other end get closer and closer to the light when it is insight. I lived in hope that I will come to find happiness down the path I paved for myself. It felt cold out in the shade waiting for the light of hope I want so much to shine down on me. Forever I do not want to be poor going through hardship, stuck in Rochdale is not where I want to be for the rest of my year's.

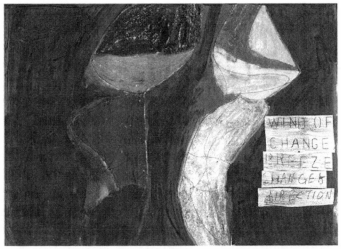

Luke and Nathan were making up and breaking up for the past few weeks, eventually their relationship had strained there was no way backing to make up so they fell out. Whenever Luke was angry, it intimidated Nathan. I think Luke's mind blew up because of the inability to cope with too many of Nathan troubles was a burden to him because of all his cares and worries. Luke took him under his wing tried to sort out his problems. Nathan felt frightened for his life when sparks flew. Since September, Nathan came knocking at my door every day. He told me that I am miserable because I did not say much to him. He told me that I am in wonderland. I felt bored whenever he came round because he distracted me from whatever it was I was doing, we just sat there listening to music. All he talked about was sex and shit. He had some kind of fixation with what you do on the toilet. He lived inside his head telling me about the times he went to the café in town and many girls wanted to have sex with him. He is so desperate he tried it on with me.

After about a month I found Nathan annoying, he became too much for me to cope with. He used to sometimes shout my name through the letterbox then go back into his own flat. I would answer the door he told me to stop knocking on his door shouting his name. I felt like having one of my drastic attacks and attacking him with a cactus plant. He came knocking on my door asking me if I would give him £2 for cigarettes. He was topless so he picked up my jumper off the stair banister and put it on. I did not give him any money because he annoyed me. I'm sure he did not really want to so why did he keep on pestering for sex but he felt so sure of him self one day he will get me into bed. He needed more to do to occupier his mind all he did was listen to music. He even asked me if I would pay for the alcoholic drinks. He insulted me by saying I am tight and miserable. He did not hurt my feelings because compared to him I am untouchable. I do not hurt when people want to hurt me.

In May, I stopped going to the education centre because my mind switched off. I felt like I could not paint anymore. For over a year I let painting take over my life I drew 461 pictures. I smashed up my glass paintings, every thing I made in pottery because I wanted to forget I ever went to that place. I saw myself back in another slump and could not find the strength to get out of it. I found the intensity unbearable not knowing when I will find my way back from the brink. The anticipation awaiting a breakthrough became unbearable. I woke up in the mornings feeling like I do not want to leave the house. Feelings of unworthiness drove me to tears. Over the years I have been reclusive and isolated, boredom drives me to tears. I felt brain-dead because of feelings of deadness in my life. Rue, Posy two new support workers and Leda kept on suggesting I should go to rubbish classes until I die. In the meantime, until I am certain about where I was heading I went out with social groups on Tuesdays and Thursdays.

My new pastime became watching musicals I brought from music stores in Manchester and Rochdale. I was able to afford to buy new clothes because I stopped buying art materials. Evan moved in to flat two in November two thousand and three. Hugo told Eve he has a four-seated sofa that is leather he might not be able to get it into his flat because the living quarters in flat two are not on ground level. He might not be able to get it up the stairs. I agreed to exchange my two sofas for his green sofa before I had seen it and a two blue-seated sofa that was already in flat two. When Hugo and Evan came knocking at my door to give me the sofa I did not like it but did not say anything. It stunk of cigarettes. In my lounge green leather sofa and a blue sofa did not match so I ripped some of it up with my bare arms. I titled the blue sofa up on its side in the kitchen corner. I sat on cousins until my new sofas were delivered I ordered from the catalogue.

Posy and Rue phoned up Amber my occupational therapist. Dr. Newton gave me medication that will to stop my depression. Since July, my ripped up sofa had been up on its side in front of the stairs. I found it back breaking squeezing past it whenever I walked up and down the stairs. I brought a saw from the hardware store, moved the sofa into the lounge and cut up the wooden framework. I put all of the upholstery into bin bags, piled the wood in the kitchen because Mr.Caneek does not like rubbish in the car park outside his restaurant; that is where the bins are.

Eventually I put all of the rubbish outside near the bins because Posy phoned the council told them to move all the rubbish. It was piled up outside for weeks. Nathan was evicted so Ebony painted his flat with Posy who also cleaned the flat; Mr. Caneek told Ebony to take the rubbish outside to the tip. A ripped up sofa was a piece of art because it was like a sculpture. Rue quit her job because she was also a hairdresser, could not fit hairdressing in with her support work. She became obsessive because all she ever talked about with me was what she wanted me to do is go to rubbish classes. Kept on saying I look fed up, go to art classes

For months every time I went into Rochdale Town Centre George Michael's music always seemed to be playing. I foresee new horizons in distance reach of him because of the picture I have drawn of a letter, which I think, is of George. I gazed out of the window into the unknown. I watched the sunrise in the east. When the line met with the earth and sky, I left house for a walk with my gown on. Out in the cold night when I could see the horizon over the ocean what it did to me is I kept on believing I will have joy in my life when I come through hard times. I felt dejected when nothing emerged through night dreams...light dreamer

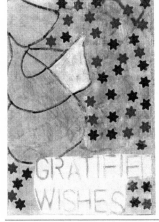

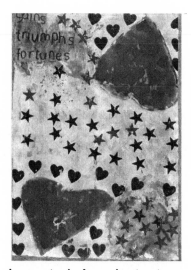

I wanted Angels to turn my grey ambience...to grey clouds so a rainbow would shine down above me. I felt as if I was lost in the wilderness in a dark horrible place. I wanted to change direction in life...but could not make it on my own to get onto a new open road. A clouded mind does not keep you grounded. It would be helpful to have somebody to be my strength and helper. I wanted to aspire to become a much more centered person. Meet my match with somebody who as a brilliant mind and greatness. I think I could measure up to somebody who has gifted creative talents. Go on holidays to the countryside and to the coast. Scattered pieces will not fall down from the cloud & earth until I know where I am heading. Inside my mind landscapes always seem to be winter. I see monsters surrounded by fire. Up in the sky I see two angels.

DARKENED LIGHT

In Rochdale, there is an employment service that specializes in helping people with mental health problems find work. Since May, I had not done anything constructive. I felt empty as if loss time is catching up with me. I became desperate for mental stimulation one of my hobbies became doing double-sided jigsaws. I needed to get on to the right open road, go in the right direction so that I will not fall into another black hole. I kept my mind focused on exhibiting my paintings. Waiting and waiting is all I ever do to get on to my gift pathway and move onto higher ground.

A big boss in high places will decide my outcome if my dreams will come true. I am not in control because that same person will decide my fate. Living inside a black hole as happened much too often in my life. When everything falls into place, everything falls into my lap I may never fall into another black hole I want to make room for growth and inner development, seize my chances when they come around. I will aspire to my aspirations. I will not stop dreaming because I will not stop believing.

My family would not want anything to do with me. I do not have a conscience so I will not miss anybody. Children forget people. I do not remember how bad it was anymore it is as if I have blocked it all out. Writing unblocked repressed feelings and emotions. My mum's sister Freya and Brother Lenny, Great Auntie June played a big part in how I grew up. Every time they saw me at their house, family celebrations always said I am like my mum, I cannot speak. It always hurt I felt like crying. They could see the pain in my eyes but would not stop insulting me. I became more and more withdrawn; all I could see with in was a spastic. I look so normal on the outside but inside I am a retard.

Floating on my cloud from every point of the compass the ocean rough and stormy I saw a star shuttling, zooming here and there, that is why I have to catch it when I reach the foreshore. When I hear the gentle ringing sound of my white precious my fallen star will shuttle into my arms, where I will catch it under the purple night sky, it will happen when the ocean is much calmer.

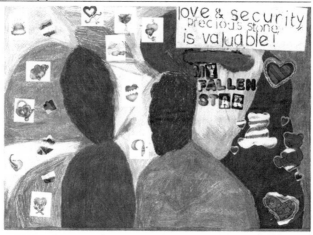

DARKENED LIGHT

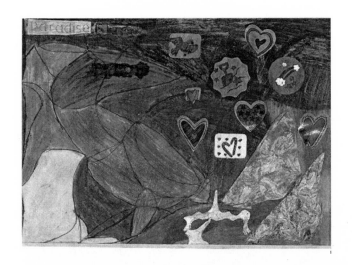

I looked into his eyes and desired a happy fate. When I fell into him, he gave his hands to hold, and then wrapped myself around him. My heartbeat fluttered just for him. Burning up, heating passions burning out of me. It was a lovely dreamy encounter when cupid arrow burst the bubble. The earth moved between us as I gave myself to him, in return he gave himself to me. We are the perfect match I think the world of him.

We fell in love listening to the sound of the symphony. We danced on air to the music. Fermenting raised my temperature. Kissed red-hot lips tasted ripe vine. Naked soft skin slept with him. We set sail together as one across the ocean to our paradise island. Life is a beach. I soaked up the warmth of the atmosphere. I floated in the shallow end of the ocean. We have a love affair with water because it is a turn on.

We headed for the hills to a magical place in the mountains.
Silver and gold ambience surrounded us.
Butterflies, Butterflies, roses fall down from the sky we slept on petals.
Fairy and gold dust floated in the air.

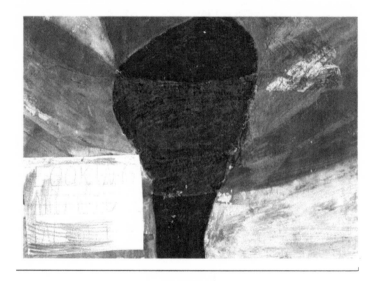

Seeing life as a journey is the glimmer of hope that has kept me going. Since 1996, my story has centered on reaching my mountain landscape. I had something to hold onto and believe into aim for. I had been living my life since two thousand two incoherent with the pictures in this chapter.

DARKENED LIGHT

He is the star that rises and falls. The light of love shined brightly in my eyes and beamd in my heart. He would brighten up my life, happiness at last be mine. My pledge to him dedicates a song to me. A letter from George is a wish I waited to long by it was hard when I thought I would not ever get to him so the time will come for me to succeed.

For year's I have not been going anywhere fast, standing at the starting post for year's waiting for.... George too discovers me so I will make it as an artist and sell pictures. All I need is for George to understand how much his music touched my life, because I believe that mountain landscape is he. Getting there is something for him to sing about, so strike up your band and play music to my ears. Scattered pieces would be a heart-rending song. Writing sentiments in a song based on my journey is news to impart to the world at large.

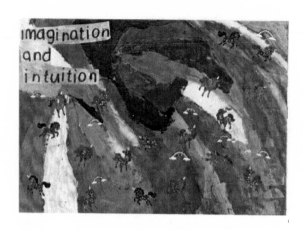

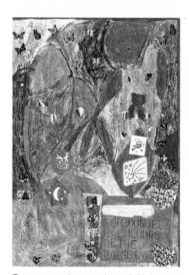

George has the Midas touch to be able to write scattered pieces. Setting myself this challenge, he is my bull's eye on target. He is the positive aspect to my current cloud. I also want George to write a musical based on my fortune journey. Scattered pieces just may be his last musical note. Writing and recording scattered pieces is my gift pathway because a change of season is like a new full moon. Atmosphere all right...told ideally. A new bench made...I thought I raked hill.

Making concrete plans would fire me up with enthusiasm. When setting my world on fire I will be full of joys of life. I want to impress him with my inspired ideas. He is my favorite....my only one, no between. I do not like anybody but him. Diverted in my chosen path, I went for gold. I hoped things would go well for me. I felt positive being the mastermind behind my great plan. I felt disenchanted embarking on a new venture. It made my journey a good deal smoother. In real life, I will know when I have reached my mountaintop and living in luxury. I will have expensive possessions. Some would say give her an almost full life.

Moving at a snails pace was worth the wait because I freed myself from constraints. Do turtles move faster than caterpillars? I do not know. Caterpillars turn into butterflies but do not fly faster than birds.

From all I have heard.
What have I learnt?
What have I done that been worth doing?
What have I done that is worth knowing?

SUSAN SPLAINE

My philosophy on life is there are too many bad apples.

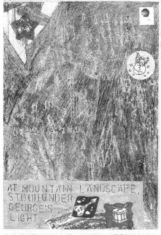

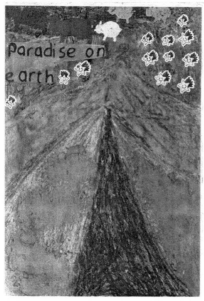

Printed in the United Kingdom
by Lightning Source UK Ltd.
126435UK00001B/2/P